KAYLEIGH PURSER is a
therapist and author.

She started her massa[
2004, where she studied hol
focusing on pain managemen
Over the years, she added more treatments, including racials and
Reiki, becoming a Reiki Master in 2018.

Kayleigh spent years working in different areas of the spa
industry, from full time spa therapist jobs to casual contracts and
agency work. Her years of experience finally led to her creating her
own temporary spa recruitment agency – Sapphire Spa Solutions
– its sole purpose, to support other self-employed therapists to
build and grow their own private practices and support their
families in a safe working environment.

After a car crash in 2013 caused severe spinal compression
and torn tendons, Kayleigh felt the need to find a means of
massage therapy that supports the health and wellbeing of the
therapist, prevents injury, and eliminates stress and exhaustion.
In 2019, The Purser Method of deep tissue massage therapy
was patented, and Kayleigh turned her attention to teaching the
method to spas and individual therapists.

Kayleigh can also be found teaching the occasional Reiki
Retreat in the Cotswolds.

Find out more about Purser Method training at:
www.pursermethod.co.uk

Join the Sapphire Team as a self-employed therapist at:
www.sapphirespasolutions.com

Follow on Instagram:
@kayleigh_pursermethod and **@sapphirespasolutions**

How Deep Should I Go?

Kayleigh
Purser

SilverWood

Published in 2021 by SilverWood Books

SilverWood Books Ltd
14 Small Street, Bristol, BS1 1DE, United Kingdom
www.silverwoodbooks.co.uk

ISBN 978-1-80042-136-3 (paperback)
ISBN 978-1-80042-137-0 (ebook)

British Library Cataloguing in Publication Data
A CIP catalogue record for this book is
available from the British Library

Page design and typesetting by SilverWood Books

To Silviu, for your unwavering support

Contents

Introduction

It has always been a dream of mine to write a book. I have started many books and they mostly remain unfinished. I have never before had the courage to try to publish one.

After creating The Purser Method of deep tissue massage therapy, I set about trying to write a serious book about my journey through my career, culminating in my discovery and development of this unique technique. After pushing myself to write the first part of the book, 2020 and COVID-19 happened, and I lost all motivation and love for the book. Every time I sat down to force more words out, I just became overwhelmed with the grief of losing the job that I loved so much.

As with all grieving processes, I came to a beautiful moment of clarity, and I realised that I am not alone and that there are thousands of massage and beauty therapists out there who are all feeling this same terrifying loss of work, income and sense of self.

After exploring those feelings further, I realised that I had lost my true sense of self a long time ago. In my desperation to appear the cool, calm, professional business owner, therapist and director of a team of other therapists, I had developed a very serious, stand-offish personality that did not belong to me. I had lost that cheeky little spark that had been my true self. The biggest reason that my previous book attempts had failed was because I was being too serious and had lost all of my 'fun'.

So, I made the decision to say, "Fuck it, this is me," and write a book that is brutally, hilariously honest about the slightly darker side of the industry that I love so much.

After a catch up over a delightful wine spritzer with the gorgeous Susie Mackie, she gave me a copy of her book, *Women of Spirit*, which I devoured over a matter of days. This book gave me the inspiration to reach out to other therapists. Susie supported my idea and even guided me through the legalities of doing this. I proceeded to reach out to therapist friends and colleagues while we were all in the same limbo of waiting to go back to work.

Chatting through everyone's unique, hilarious and occasionally disturbing stories was the highlight of COVID-19 lockdown for me. I have never laughed so much! Being able to write these stories has been an absolute privilege and I am honoured to be able to share them with you now alongside one or two of my own.

Many of the therapists have decided to remain anonymous.

To protect the identity of therapists, clients and businesses, no names or locations have been given to any of these stories.

My one stipulation with every therapist that I have had the pleasure of speaking to is that the story they share absolutely has to be REAL.

This ALL happened!

Part One

Lessons in Hygiene

Feet; some people love them, some people hate them but wherever you stand, there is no denying that no one wants to touch feet that haven't been washed in days, in the height of summer!

I had a client once that smelt so bad, I struggled to be in the same room as him. When I pulled back the towel to start the massage, the towel was slightly stuck to his skin from all the dirt on his back.

I cannot imagine the number of times in the summer months that I have massaged clients who have just had a spray tan and I end up with orange hands and arms! They don't seem to realise that tan comes off with oil and there is nothing we can do about it.

In Very Poor Taste

I have had a vast and varied career in massage therapy. For a short time, in the very early days, I was working with a team of mobile massage therapists, going into hotels that did not have any spa facilities and offering treatments within the guest's room. I admit, it is not the highlight of my career. Those massage couches are damned heavy and when you add in all the towels and products that you have to carry around, it gets pretty cumbersome and more than slightly back breaking. The pay was good, but not amazing, considering the level of inconvenience and travel. You might be called to a hotel in the middle of the Cotswolds for just one back, neck and shoulder massage and then expected to drive for up to an hour to the next hotel in the arse end of nowhere for an Indian head massage, and by the time you're home, that's taken four plus hours out of your day and all for just £30! So, in hindsight, it was actually crap pay.

I was getting towards the end of my time doing this sort of work and I was really starting to feel fed up with it all. The number of innuendos you have to deal with, the occasional times you feel incredibly unsafe around a person, locked in their hotel room with them, or the times when you are massaging a person and being closely observed by their partner, lying on the hotel bed doing goodness knows what under the covers was really starting to wear thin.

I arrived at one of my favourite hotels in one of the most beautiful, picturesque villages of the Cotswolds on a slightly soggy spring afternoon. Hulking my massive massage couch, with towels, oils and everything stuffed into the carry case, making it weigh in at around sixteen to eighteen kilograms, I gingerly mounted the stone steps up to the hotel entrance. I arrived at the reception desk to be informed that, unfortunately, there were no team members available to help me to get the couch up the stairs – not that it made much of a difference to normal. I was often too proud and/or stubborn to let anyone help me with my couch anyway.

The receptionist smiled brightly and declared, "It's OK, though, you're just up the first flight of stairs, first door on the right."

At least it was just the one flight of stairs this time. I started thinking that maybe it wasn't so bad after all. I had a full body massage booked in, which is an hour and fifteen minutes and would pay me £35. It was my only booking for the whole day and it had taken forty-five minutes to get to the hotel, but it was a Saturday so at least it meant having most of the weekend off work for a change.

I knocked carefully on the door and a white-haired gentleman answered in shirt and smart trousers. Now I am pretty terrible at guessing people's ages, but I would have put him at around late fifties to early sixties. Very respectable looking and polite. I didn't feel at all uncomfortable with him and I was right at the top of the stairs anyway; if I ran out of the room and looked over the bannister, I would be looking straight down at the top of the receptionist's head. I didn't think I had anything at all to fear here so I began to relax and get my couch set up. I politely told him that it would take me a few minutes to get set up, I confirmed his treatment with him and gave him a consultation form to fill out, which he took into the en suite bathroom with him to get ready for his treatment. I set up my couch, with towels, couch roll and oils ready on the side with couch roll underneath to stop any spills on any of the furniture. I set up some music and I waited. And waited.

After a while, I started to get a bit concerned, so I gently called out that I was all set up and ready to start his treatment. He called back that he would just be a moment. There were some odd grunts and noises from the bathroom and then the shower came on. Now I was starting to get a bit annoyed. I had agreed to meet a friend after work and I get extremely agitated if I ever run late. I must have already been waiting for around ten minutes and he had just got in the shower! I felt really angry that he was wasting my time, I had arrived early to make sure I had set up time, I had been ready to go at the start time of the treatment and now he was getting in the shower, well he was definitely having a shorter treatment. For a lousy £35 I was not going to over run on my treatment time! The shower stopped and there were more grunts and mutterings. Maybe this guy was older than I thought?

Eventually, a very unsure voice asked, "Is it OK if I come out just in my towel robe?"

Being very twitchy about time, I just called back, "Yes, that's fine," not thinking about the underwear situation.

He came out of the bathroom looking very nervous and unsure. I thought that maybe this was a new situation for him and that he either wasn't used to having massages or he wasn't used to having them in a hotel room setting. I therefore thought it would be wise to ask him if he wished for me to leave the room while he got onto the couch.

He looked very relieved and said, "Yes, I will call when I am ready."

So I stepped outside the room to wait, again.

I had a little peek over the balcony and down at reception, just to be sure that someone was still there. The receptionist was on the phone. And I waited.

I wondered if perhaps I had not heard him, so I put my ear up to the door and edged the door open a tiny bit. I softly called, "Are you ready?"

My answer was not a voice but a soft, yet very audible fart, one of those ones that lasts for a few seconds with a slight squeak at the end. I desperately tried not to laugh.

Eventually, he replied, "Yes, you can come in."

I took a deep breath (outside of the room), composed myself and stepped in. He was lying face down with the towel covering him. I asked if he was comfortable and checked his form for anything that I needed to be aware of. I also asked him to clarify if there was anything that I needed to be aware of – allergies, aches, pains, etc. or areas he wished for me to concentrate on.

He replied, "I have been feeling a little out of sorts and run down so a relaxing and very gentle massage please." He really emphasised the gentle, so I started with my breathing exercises and pulled back the towel. Of course, there were no pants or boxers for me to tuck the towel into, but never mind, I did not have any unsafe feelings about this client at all.

I started my massage treatment, warming up the muscles gently and doing my own rhythmic deep breathing to keep my movements slow and gentle. I always breathe through my nose when I am treating – I feel that it helps to keep me focused and slow. It may have been a mistake.

His back was so tense, and I really felt like I needed to add more pressure, but he had been so adamant about a gentle massage. I checked with him and he said the pressure was good. After a while, he did start to relax into the treatment. His breathing became deeper and I wondered if he was falling asleep. All of a sudden, his lower back tensed up and his whole body started to stiffen. I thought perhaps I had shocked him or maybe had gone deeper than I had intended. Then another soft, wispy fart came out. Then another, and another.

He muttered an apology and I said, "Don't worry, it happens when you are relaxed."

But the smell, oh my God! It was like something had died and my eyes were actually watering.

A more alarming trump erupted from his arse, which made me almost buckle over trying to restrain my laugh. My belly ached with the unspilled laughter, my eyes streamed, and I couldn't decide if I wanted to breathe through my nose or my mouth and risk tasting it! The next one came out like a bloody trumpet announcing a royal occasion and I thought I would retch. I think the couch actually vibrated and the towel definitely moved. I was now crying, trying desperately not to breathe or laugh and still trying to give a gentle, relaxing massage. Then arrived the most disturbing one of all, the one that sounds wet and dangerous and he urgently said, "I'm not feeling too well," and asked me to leave.

I mumbled something about the time, and he said, "I'll pay for the whole treatment. Please go."

I barely made it out of the room when he leapt off the couch like a spring rabbit and ran into the bathroom.

I gave it a moment for some of the fog to clear, took a gulp of air from the hallway and stepped back in to retrieve my towels, couch and belongings. I gave a cordial call towards the bathroom to say that I was packing up and would be gone soon and that the fee would be added to his hotel bill, he shouted back, "That's fine, just go."

I packed away as quickly as I possibly could. Just as I was reaching the door to leave, the most atrocious sound came from the bathroom, followed by a mournful moan and a string of curses. I managed to make it back to the car before I howled with laughter.

Romance in the Spa

We have all had those clients who are a little, how should I say it...vocal, during their massage treatments. The moaners and groaners and occasionally the guttural screamers! So, it isn't all that unusual in a spa to hear slightly sexual sounding moaning coming from one of the treatment rooms. I came out of the little bathroom next to my treatment room to have the beautiful silence of the treatment room corridors broken by just such a sound. Not thinking much of it, I went back into my room to change towels and clean up after my last client. I took the towels to the laundry room and on my way back passed by the couples' treatment room and Rasul Mud room. The moaning noises were still going on, a little bit louder now, and I realised they were coming from the couples' room. I had a little giggle to myself as I imagined my poor colleagues in there trying not to feel uncomfortable or giggle to each other while this was going on.

Shaking my head, I couldn't help but think which client was making the noise and what on earth was their partner thinking while they were making all of these sounds?!

Back in my room, I wiped down the couch and laid out fresh towels. I had a bit of a break between clients, so I enjoyed the moment of calm and took my time with my tidying. Deciding to top up the massage oils, I headed out to the prep room. The two therapists that I knew were working in the couples' room were in the prep room when I went in.

I made a remark about their noisy clients, "Which client was making all that noise? How did you keep a straight face?"

The girls looked at each other, a bit puzzled. "We haven't started the massage yet, we have only done the scrub, they're in the mud room now."

"Then who was moaning?" I asked.

The three of us exchanged a look and then all headed back to the treatment rooms to see if there were still any noises. Sure enough, we could hear loud moaning coming from the room, but now it was clearly two voices, male and female. *Oh my God*, my colleagues mouthed at me, one gestured to the Rasual Mud room door. We each crept towards the door and leaned our ears closer to it. The two therapists made exaggerated faces and pointed wildly at the door. *I know!* I mouthed back.

We headed back to the prep room and shut the door.

"Oh my God, oh my God, oh my God!" one of the therapists said.

"Are they having sex in the mud room?" the other exclaimed.

"What is wrong with people, what do we do?"

"I don't know, urgh, who DOES that?"

"They're staying in the hotel; they HAVE a room!"

"What do we do?"

"We have to tell the manager," I said, "surely that's a bloody health and safety risk!"

"Oh my God, we are going to have to clean that up!" one therapist wailed.

"Oh, hell no," said the other and stormed out to find the manager.

After a while, we headed back out to the treatment room corridor to see what was happening. The head receptionist was with the other therapist leaning close to the Rasul Mud room. There were still noises going on in there.

"This has happened before; I can't believe some people!" said the head receptionist, "I should sound the bloody alarm in there, are there any other treatments going on right now?"

"Yeah, room one and four are in use, I'm not sure when they finish."

"I'm heading back into treatment soon," I said.

"We still have to do their massages," one therapist looked down at her feet in defeat.

"Oh no, they can leave without their treatment, this is unacceptable," said the head receptionist.

Relief washed over the two therapists' faces, "We'll still have to clean up after them though." The relief was short lived.

I checked the time on my watch and realised I would need to collect my client from reception soon. I left the girls debating how to get the clients out of the mud room and headed back to prep to top up my oils and get ready for my treatment.

I collected my client and took him through to the treatment room. I went through his consultation and explained the treatment to him. I left to give him privacy to get ready for the treatment. When I came out of the room, I watched as the head therapist frog marched two very sheepish looking clients out of the Rasul Mud room and out towards the changing rooms. Her face was a picture of silent rage! The two therapists were stood outside the couples' room doors looking like they didn't know if they should laugh or cry.

"Oh my God, she is so mad with them, I've never seen her angry before," one therapist said about the head receptionist.

"I still can't believe people would think it was OK to have sex in a Rasul!" I said.

"I know," exclaimed the other therapist, "I mean, can you imagine the infection you could get if you got clay stuck up THERE?" she pointed animatedly at her fanny.

We all giggled as I headed back to my room to start my treatment, hoping that this one wouldn't be a moaner!

Just Having a Crack

I would say, as a general rule, I am pretty relaxed about my treatments and my interactions with my clients and we do very often have a chat and a giggle. Especially with new clients, I find that a little humour helps to break any nervous tension and I quickly build up a good rapport with my patients. I appreciate that it is a very private and personal thing having a massage treatment, and I respect and am grateful for the trust that my clients put in me.

I once had a treatment room set up in the downstairs office at my home address. You came through the front door and there it was on your left. This meant that clients didn't need to go through the house, and it felt private enough and cut off from my living space to give me that break between work and home. I used to love it; it was so much more convenient than renting a room in a salon at that point in my career.

As I was working from home, I was a bit more selective about my clients and didn't give my home address out to just anyone. Therefore, all of my clients either knew me personally or we had friends in common. This, in my mind, ruled out any unfortunate incidents, kept me safe from those odd clients who seem to confuse massage therapy with something a little more lewd and only brought me clients who would be respectful and well presented.

This set up had been working very well for me for over two years and I was feeling very relaxed and comfortable with the steady clientele that I had. I was very blessed to have mostly regular clients who often referred their family and friends to me, so I rarely had to advertise or invite new people into the house. It was perfect. I had developed close relationships with most of my clients and we would often chat before, during and after treatments. Working from home gave me the enviable position of being able to have as long a gap as I wanted between clients and I would very often book extra 'clean up' time after certain people so that we could have a cup of tea and a gossip after their treatment.

One such client was a family friend, a very lovely woman who had been seeing me since before I set up in the house. She had referred her sister, daughter, husband and a few friends to me over the years and most of them had become regular clients. I trusted her judgement implicitly and would still consider her to be a very good friend to this day.

After a treatment we sat drinking herbal tea and making small talk and she mentioned a work colleague of hers that was in need of some help with her back. "Her posture is just awful and it's making her hunch over. She's in terrible pain!

"I was telling her all about you, you know. She couldn't believe that I see you every month! She must think I'm terribly posh now!" We laughed.

"Can I send her to you? She really needs your magic hands!"

Well, I couldn't refuse such flattery and everyone that she had previously sent over was delightful, so I readily agreed, and a few days later I had the inevitable phone call and plea for help from her colleague. This woman was suffering terribly with pain in her shoulders and lower back. She thought it was most likely posture related as she had always had bad posture, and working long hours at a computer was not helping. She was aware that she should be taking regular breaks but wasn't doing so and very often had her lunch at her desk, still slumped over the keyboard or with the phone cradled between her ear and right shoulder. She clearly needed some help and so we discussed potential treatment plans for her and made arrangements for an initial treatment. We agreed a date and time and I gave her all the relevant details and a consultation form to fill out and send back or print out and bring with her on the day.

The day came and I answered the door to a very lovely woman, a lot younger than I had expected for someone with the ailments she had described. She was in her early forties, quite tall (which wouldn't help her posture) and reasonably slender. I have to admit, I was expecting someone overweight to account for some of her difficulties so I was a little surprised. Whilst standing, she looked fairly straight backed, a little curve to the upper spine but nothing terrible and her right shoulder was definitely lower than her left. As soon as she sat down, though, she almost bent over, her shoulders slumped and she almost collapsed into the chair. The poor thing just looked exhausted.

We had our initial consultation chat and I got to know a bit more about her, she was very open and witty. She had a very strong work ethic and seemed to be pushing herself a little too hard but otherwise her lifestyle was quite healthy. We confirmed what was needed from the treatment and I exited the treatment room for her to get ready for a back, neck and shoulder massage.

As I entered the room, I had to smile. It was almost military neat the way she had folded and placed her clothes, shoes, bag and jewellery. Even the towel covering her was perfectly neat and tidy, no adjustments needed at all. I definitely liked this client!

I always begin treatments with a good stretch over the towels and a little trigger pointing work if necessary. She was so tense and tight that I spent a little longer on this than I would usually do and tried to focus in on the pressure points to help her body to relax. Working my way from feet to scalp, I pressed and stretched as much as I could, gently rolling and lifting her hips and shoulders. Leaning as much of my weight into her as I could and checking pressures with her, I worked my way around her body through the towels, lightly palpating and pummelling where needed. Her breathing became deeper and her muscles started to relax into the rhythm of my stretches. The music had a soft, lilting pulse to it and I timed my moves to this, both of us getting deeper into this relaxing treatment.

My treatments are all very intuitive so I never do the same one twice. I instinctively knew that it was now time to move into a contact treatment and I very gently pulled back the towel. Her underwear was very high, so I tucked the towel around her knickers and gently started to manoeuvre them down to expose her lower back and the tops of her glutes. I was still in my zen flow and it took me a moment to notice the smell. I had mostly had my eyes closed or quite unfocused, as I usually do in treatments, but this smell made my eyes snap right open. I was looking directly at the top of the crack of her backside and I think I noticed the knickers first, with my lovely white towels tucked into them and the unmistakeable signs of skid marks.

I felt myself recoiling but it was a bit too late – my beautiful towels were indeed tucked into her skiddy underpants and I had wiped the towel down the top of her backside. To my horror, I could still see a long smear of poop in the crack of her backside and slightly above.

I was about halfway through her allotted time and I had completely lost my flow. I very carefully pulled the now ruined towel back up over the poo marks, luckily hiding the worst of the smell, and continued with her treatment, doing my best to stay with the rhythm of the music and not think about the state of my towels…

After she left, I threw the towel in the bin.

Part Two

The Good, the Bad and the Bloody Clueless

I have a lovely client who loves herbal teas. When I started offering herbal teas at the end of my treatments, she started sending me a tea bag in the post every time she tried something new that she thought I would like.

I worked in a spa a while ago that used to have duvets on the beds to keep the clients warm. I used to think it was a really lovely idea, especially for when men would fall asleep face up on the couch and then things might start to accidentally rise – it's less embarrassing for them when there is a duvet there to hide it. I changed my mind after I had a client jerk himself off under the duvet, whilst watching me working!

"What do you mean by Complementary Therapist?"

"I work alongside other healthcare professionals."

"Oh right, I thought you just meant that your job was to compliment people."

Which Way to Turn

The number of therapists who have contacted me to share their stories and have mentioned a client who has faced the wrong way for a treatment is just too numerous to mention. I have completely lost count of the number of times that I have heard about it, experienced it myself or had therapists write to me about it. I could not put all of these stories into one book or it would fill it!

I am not sure where the miscommunication comes from, especially when the therapist says before the treatment starts, please lie face up on the couch, or please lie on your stomach under this towel to start your treatment. Also, the number of times that therapists say to a client, cover yourself with this towel, and then the client lies on top of it or throws it on the floor. I once had a client hang the towel that I had asked them to use to cover themselves over with on the back of the door and then strip off completely and lie on their back on the couch facing the ceiling, for a back massage!

I digress! I had to pick just one of the stories that I was sent regarding the which way to face phenomena, and this one has to be my very favourite…

Over the years I have had many clients struggle with getting onto the massage couch, whether it is that they get caught up in the towel or they can't seem to cover themselves over with it, they face the wrong way or they take every scrap of clothing off when you expressly ask them to keep underwear on or they just stand awkwardly next to the couch because they have forgotten everything that you asked them to do. As a result of this, with all of my patients, I always ask them if they want me to leave the room while they are getting ready or if they are comfortable with me just lifting the towel up for them so that they can easily get onto the couch. It is very rare that any client now asks me to leave the room. So, I usually have a bit more control of the situation and am actually on hand to direct if the client is unsure how to lie for their treatment.

On this occasion, I am not sure if the fault was mine or my client's and I will leave that for you to decide. I have racked my brains for days after this incident trying to figure out if I said the wrong thing, assumed the wrong thing or if my client was just on another planet!

Firstly, I think it is important to point out that this was not a new client. This was someone who I had seen many times beforeat the same venue, on the same couch, for the same treatment.

Secondly, my couch is an electric, bifold couch (the head can be raised and so can the feet) with a detachable horseshoe face cradle and I always have the face cradle attached at one end and the feet raised slightly for support at the opposite end.

As always, I offered to leave if my client wished for privacy despite knowing that she had never asked me to leave before. As expected, she declined. I stood to the side of the couch with the

34

face cradle to my left and the bottom of the couch (with the raised footrest) to my right. I lifted the towel so that I could not see my client getting changed, to give her privacy and so that when she was ready, she could lie straight down on the couch. I am ninety-nine per cent sure that I said, "When you are ready, please lie face down on the couch." Perhaps I did not. It is possible that, because she had been so many times before, I didn't feel the need to tell her how to lie down.

I think this is the right time to point out the third thing – the client was booked to have a back massage.

I could hear my client approach the couch and I looked to my left at the face cradle expecting to see the back of her head, indicating that she was on the couch and that I could lower the towel. My arms were starting to ache a bit from holding the towel up for so long. It was winter so I assumed that she had a lot of layers to take off. I was surprised to see the soles of her feet instead. So, I quickly said, "I'm sorry, you need to have your face in the cradle, could you turn around please."

She apologised and her feet disappeared, only to shortly reappear again, this time toes pointing up.

Once again, I said, "I'm sorry, please could you have your face in the cradle, you're the wrong way around."

"Oops, I'm sorry, silly me," came the reply, followed by the disappearance of the feet and some more huffing and puffing.

Then the client's face appeared. She was lying face up on the couch, at least at the right end this time but the wrong way around.

I smiled down at her, "I'm so sorry but I thought we were doing a back massage, I need you to be lying face down, please."

She smiled back at me and giggled. She got up, and then her bloody feet appeared again!

At this point, my arms were absolutely killing me from holding the towel up and I had to lower the towel down. "This isn't very comfortable," she said. No shit, I was thinking, but instead smiled and calmly said, "Your face needs to be in the face cradle, in the hole, here." I pointed to where her feet were.

"Oopsie, silly me," she said, giggling. "You can tell I need this today."

I lifted the towel up and waited for her to turn around.

Her face appeared again, looking up at me from the face cradle. I dropped the towel over her and sighed. I could not hide the frustration in my voice.

"You need to get off the couch," I said. "I can't work on your back when you are lying on it. Let me show you."

I left the towel draped over her and let her get up, holding the towel around herself.

I then climbed onto the couch the way that she should have done.

"Oh, I see," she said, "the lump at the end of the couch confused me."

I got up off the couch and helped her to lie down and arranged the towel over her. "That's for your feet, so there is less pressure on your back," I said.

"Oh, that makes sense now, you don't normally have that."

Somehow, I managed to stop myself from saying, it is ALWAYS like that! And I started the massage.

Laughter Is the Best Medicine

It has been quite therapeutic, and very enjoyable, looking back at my funny spa moments. It feels good to reminisce. One memory in particular got me really smiling so I thought it would be the best one to share.

I was working as an agency therapist, popping in and out of different spas, all with different clientele, atmospheres and procedures. Each spa was different from the last and it really kept you on your toes remembering and managing the expectations of each one. Some were more laid back than others, the clientele maybe being a bit more brash and noisy, whereas others might be very posh, strict and very, very quiet. Wherever you go, you always treat the place as if it is a five-star award winning exclusive spa with very strict, professional guidelines. This particular spa was exactly like that!

I was working a really hectic shift, my schedule (and everyone else's) was jam packed all day. There was no room for error, running late or getting caught up chatting with a client. The spa rules were strictly professional, and noise had to be kept to an absolute minimum. There had been complaints from that spa about an agency staff closing a cupboard door too loudly during a treatment! I guess you can understand, when it's such a busy day and all of the treatment rooms are full, the last thing you want is to be able to hear someone else banging around in the room next door.

All of my clients that day had been very well to do and almost a bit snobby. I remember going out to the lounge to collect one of my clients. She was very well presented, probably in her mid-sixties and very posh! I greeted her politely in the lounge, where she had been sitting with her friends. I wasn't sure if they had been drinking a little as they were all quite jolly and excitable. I took her through to the treatment room, trying to be as quiet as I could as we walked past the other occupied rooms, but she was quite giddy and didn't seem to notice my whispering and hushed tones, instead being a bit more boisterous than I expected from her otherwise sophisticated appearance.

In the treatment room, I explained the procedure and went through her consultation form and then gave her a few minutes privacy to get changed while I filed the form away in the office. The massage that she was having started with a full body scrub and shower and so I had laid out disposable pants for her to wear and set out everything that would be needed for the shower, including an extra pair of disposable pants and a shower cap in case she wanted to keep her hair dry. I had explained all of this to her and shown her where everything was before I had left the room for her to get ready. I started the treatment with the body scrub and we did chat a little through this but I tried to keep my tone hushed and she was starting to unwind and lower her voice as well. When I finished the scrub, I explained to her that I would leave the room so that she could get in the shower and whilst she was in there, I would come back in to lay fresh sheets on the bed.

I also told her that there was a fresh towel to dry herself with and a shower cap if she wanted to keep her hair dry, as well as a fresh pair of the same disposable underwear she was wearing so she could have a dry pair on for her massage. I advised her to get back onto the massage couch when she had finished with her shower and that I would then come back in for her massage. I lowered the couch and waited outside for her to get into the shower.

I was listening out for the sounds of the water running so I would know when to go back in and change the towels, but instead of water, all I could hear was a loud shriek of laughter and her very posh voice shouting, "Is this shower cap meant to have holes in? Oh fuck! I think I've just put the pants back on my head!" She continued howling laughter and then shouted out again, "Oh fuck, I picked up the wrong thing, my hair is getting wet through the holes," followed by more laughter!

Before I could get back into the room to ask her to quieten down, one of the other therapists came out of her treatment room to see what was going on. I was sure she was going to be very angry with me and would report me to the agency but instead she started laughing and covering her mouth to try and keep quiet. I think I was in too much shock and panic to be able to laugh with her!

I gently knocked on the door and entered, ready to change the towels, but she was stood next to the couch wrapped in a towel pointing at the giant disposable pants on her head, still laughing and saying, "I think I may have put the wrong item on my head?" She then pulled open one of the large leg holes, revealing her soaking wet hair. She looked quite tragic and I couldn't help but laugh with her.

"Yep, you need to wear those for the next part of your treatment. I'll just change these towels and get you a fresh pair." I could see that the shower cap (still in its box and labelled SHOWER CAP) had been moved off the fresh towel that she was now wrapped in and put on the massage bed. She saw me looking at it and laughed again. "Typical me, I always get everything wrong; I should have stayed at home with the horses, I'm less of a liability there!"

I returned with fresh disposable pants, which I think she managed to rip putting on, and finished her massage treatment, both of us still smiling! When finished, I gave her the relevant after care advice and showed her back to the relaxation room to meet back up with her friends. She was still laughing and said, "I really enjoyed that treatment, and all of our laughing. I needed that, thank you!"

"Oh, I thought that was you!" one of her friends laughed. "Really, we can't take you anywhere!"

I politely took my leave saying, "Have a fantastic day, ladies" as I headed back to the treatment room to tidy up.

Too Small for Deep Tissue

I had been covering mostly massage treatments all day at a spa, it was approaching the end of the day and I had just one client left to treat. The diary said deep tissue massage, which I had mostly been doing that day. I was getting a little tired and the air-con had stopped working in the treatment rooms, so I was not feeling my best, or particularly fresh! I went to the waiting area to collect my client, a reasonably large man, around 6ft tall and broad shouldered. He was the only person in the waiting area, so I spoke as I approached him, "Are you waiting for a massage treatment?"

He looked up and without smiling said, "Yes, an hour massage."

I smiled at him and introduced myself. "I'll be your therapist today. Are you ready to come through for your treatment?"

Still no sign of a smile – in fact, he actually looked even more cross. He sighed deeply. "Well, I booked a deep tissue massage."

"Yes sir, are you ready to come through?" I tried to smile back.

"You can't do a deep tissue massage," he stated, and crossed his arms over his chest.

I rocked back on my heels slightly. I have had to deal with rude clients before, but I had never had my abilities brought to question in this manner.

"I am a trained sports massage therapist, sir," I replied. I think I had lost the smile.

"That's very good, but I did make it clear to reception that I would need a deep tissue massage and I am a big guy. You can't be expected to do a deep massage on me." I softened a little, thinking maybe he was just genuinely concerned.

"Oh, I'm sure it will be fine sir, I have worked with rugby players and alike. I have been doing this for a few years now. Are you ready to come through?"

He begrudgingly stood up and muttered under his breath. He followed me through to the treatment room and I went through his consultation form and explained the treatment. I explained that for the deep tissue massage it was up to him what areas of the body we focused on and he requested to work on just his back and the backs of his legs. He said that he got regular massages from a physiotherapist on his upper back and shoulders and didn't think that I would have the strength to deal with the knots in those areas. Rather than argue with him, I suggested that we start with his legs and work our way to his back, neck and shoulders.

I left the room to allow him to get ready.

Standing outside the room, I could feel my heart rate increasing as I decided that I really didn't like this guy. I did my best to get into my zone and slow my breathing down.

I went back into the room to start his treatment. As always, I carried out the welcome ritual with hot mitts on his feet and pressure points to the souls of his feet and around his ankles.

Rather than relax, he asked me what I thought I was doing. I explained the ritual and brought it to a swift end.

Starting his massage with his left leg, I began with long effleurage strokes with my forearm. I had barely managed two strokes when he said, "I did say deep tissue."

I apologised, tried to explain that I was just warming the muscles up, but he uttered another dismissive whatever.

Balancing my breath and trying to recentre myself, I adjusted my stance to get a deeper pressure and continued. He let out a grunt and I asked if the pressure was OK. "Yes, yes," he muttered.

I continued the treatment, not finding the levels of tension that he had led me to expect but still working with a reasonable depth. After a while, and a couple more grunts, he said, "I would like a relaxing massage." He had not mentioned this before so I just agreed and slowed down my treatment whilst still trying to deliver the pressure that he had requested. He carried on grunting and I asked again if the pressure was alright. "You are hurting me," he blurted out, and I immediately apologised and readjusted the pressure. "I want deep tissue," he shouted. I apologised again and gently reminded him that there were other treatments taking place in the rooms next door and if he could keep his voice low. I once again readjusted, trying to get deeper but without causing the pain he had mentioned.

I came to the end of the first leg and moved onto his right leg. Trying to keep myself centred, deliver a deep, but not too deep, relaxing massage and not lose my temper with the most awkward client I think I had ever had was a challenge, but I focused on my breath and carried on. This time he made no noises and after a while, started to snore. This made me smile and feel a lot more relaxed. I carried on with his treatment, covered his leg back over and moved on to his back.

I was already massaging his back when he suddenly stopped snoring and shouted, "You haven't finished my leg massage."

I apologised and gently pointed out that he had been asleep. I also reminded him that there were other treatments going on and to keep the volume down. I pointed out that we didn't have that long left for the massage, and asked if he wanted me to continue with his back or go back to his leg. He mumbled another whatever and I carried on.

I was still using forearms and a little bit of elbows around his upper back and shoulders. He grunted again, and I asked if the pressure was alright for him.

"What are you doing?" he shouted. "What are you using to massage me?"

"I'm using my forearms, sir, as you requested a deep tissue massage."

"Well, I prefer girls to massage me with their fingers." This comment made me cringe a little but I held my composure.

"I cannot get the right depth with just fingers, sir. You asked for a deep tissue massage and the best way to deliver that is with forearms and elbows."

"Why can't you use fingers?" he demanded.

"Well, in all honesty, sir, my hands and wrists have been injured in the past and deep tissue massage requires more depth. We use our forearms here to prevent injuries."

"Oh, I'm sorry that they gave me an injured therapist," he mumbled.

"I am not currently injured, sir, It's just that there have been injuries in the past from massaging with just fingers and thumbs, so we have adopted forearm massage for deep tissue. If you prefer, I will use just hands and fingers but I might not be able to provide enough pressure."

He issued another whatever and I continued with just hands and fingers.

"Ouch, you're hurting me," he shouted. I had barely touched a knot in his shoulder. I explained that I had found a knot in his shoulder and asked if he would like me to work on it.

"Yes, yes, I asked for deep tissue, get it out," he yelled.

I continued to manipulate the knot with my fingers as he had requested. He continued to yell and complain that I was hurting him.

I was completely confused and not sure what to do any more.

"If I use my forearms for this knot, I might be able to remove it with less discomfort than with my fingers. Would you like me to try, sir?"

"Yes, yes, whatever you think," he shouted.

I had barely touched him when he yelled again that I was hurting him.

I still had ten minutes left of his treatment but I just couldn't do any more.

"I'm sorry, sir, but I don't think that I am suited as your therapist. I think it's best that I stop this treatment now," I said.

"I think that's best, don't you?" he shouted back at me. I didn't bother asking him to keep his voice down, I just needed to get out of the room. I forced myself to smile politely and apologised again as he left the room. When he had gone, I let myself back into the room and let out a little cry. After a few tears, I composed myself, tidied up the room and prepared to go down to the reception to tell the manager what had happened and explain my side of it.

As I was leaving the room, the manager came up to see me. She gently guided me back into the treatment room, shutting the door behind her. Before I could say anything, she turned around and whispered, "What an asshole."

Feeling relieved, I explained my side of things and then she filled me in on what happened when he came downstairs.

"I don't know what he wanted. He said that he had booked a deep tissue massage and was angry that we had provided a therapist who was not strong enough to deliver a deep tissue massage and then complained that you had hurt him. I mean, what the fuck does he want? I pointed out that deep tissue massage often does hurt, which he agreed with and then complained that it wasn't relaxing enough!"

"Well, at one point he was snoring," I said.

My manager laughed, and said, "I don't know how you managed to spend that long in the same room as him. I wanted to punch him after a minute!"

Apparently, he was given a fifty per cent refund because he didn't get his full treatment. As far as I am aware, he did not come back for a treatment, or at least he certainly didn't come back to see me!

Knot in the Office

I was working full time at a beautiful, five-star hotel spa in the middle of the Cotswolds. Our main clientele tended to be people on business trips or visiting the area for the horse racing seasons. We tended to either be rushed off our feet with bookings or very quiet; there was never anything in between. I remember it being one of the quieter days, so I would assume that it was not race season, and as a result I was working both treatments and spa reception that day.

The other therapists must have been in treatments when an American gentleman came to the spa reception desk. He was staying in the hotel just for that night and would be leaving early in the morning, but he wanted to have a massage treatment before he left. He wanted to book a fifty-five-minute full body massage but the only way to fit him in was to tag him onto the end of my day just before I finished.

When he came back for his treatment, he told me that he was going to have to go on a conference call and he wanted me to massage him while he was on the call. I would normally find this quite odd, but I thought that it was just a matter of bad timing and that he wouldn't be able to change the time of the call. As it was the end of the day, I knew that there weren't any other treatments going on at the time of his so his call wouldn't disturb any other clients, and I said that it was fine.

I left the room to let him get ready for his treatment and when I came back in, he was lying face down on the treatment couch with his phone placed close to his head and was already on the conference call. I didn't think I should make any noise so I didn't say anything when I started the treatment. I couldn't check pressure with him or ask him to take three breaths or any of the usual welcome ritual that I would normally do. I just had to try and be as quiet as I could.

I don't think that the video was on – if it was, it would have just been showing the ceiling, but there was a big group of people on the call, which made me feel really nervous and I was so worried about making noise. The whole meeting was about organising a new contract and went on for a long time. I'm fairly sure I should not have been privy to any of the information that they were discussing so I tried not to listen in too much.

The worst part was trying not to make any sounds at all whilst doing the treatment. My treatments are usually more deep tissue than relaxing and I'm not the most graceful of therapists. I'm usually quite clumsy, so I was desperately trying to tip toe around and keep quiet. I was also a bit reluctant to use my full strength for his treatment, as the plan was to keep as quiet as possible. Unfortunately, at times, I do not know my own strength and at one point I hit a particularly big knot in his shoulder and he let out quite a moaning grunt, which made more than one of the men on the call stop and ask, "What was that?" The problem is that once you have found a knot, it's not easy to let it go and it does need to come out, but again I tried not to put too much pressure on and eased the knot as gently as I possibly could. Still, he ended up with a bit of a gasp, followed by another query on the call, "Who is that?!" I decided it was probably best to leave the shoulder alone, and carried on with my treatment as quietly as I could.

Getting him to turn over was quite tricky. He was still on the call when I needed him to turn, so I was having to whisper and tap him on the shoulder. I could hear a dog occasionally barking on the phone, so I guessed that not everyone was in an office and some people were working from home, which made me think that maybe this wasn't too unorthodox. (This was before the COVID-19 crisis when it was unusual for people to be working from home!)

He turned over and carried on chattering away on the call while I tried to tip toe around the couch again. Luckily, the call ended before the end of the treatment, so I didn't have to whisper and casually bugger off and leave him at the end. I had been a bit worried about how I was going to do that, it's not like the couches are quiet when you lower them or sit them forward!

I left the room as normal and gave him time to get ready. He still had use of the facilities so he would have gone back into the spa and probably got changed in the changing rooms downstairs. I can't remember how long it was, but I met him back at reception downstairs when he was ready to leave and he came through a bit flustered and said that his boss had just complained that people were not on the call properly and had not been at their desks the whole time. I mentioned to him that I had heard a dog barking at one point, and he looked at me pointedly and said, "Did you? Are you sure?" I confirmed that I had definitely heard something, and he shouted, "Right!" and stormed off. I still hadn't checked him out of the spa at this point, so I wasn't sure what was going on!

Outside he paced up and down in front of the spa doors whilst on the phone. He looked very animated and like he was having an argument with someone. I'm not sure if he was telling someone off or defending himself for his occasional grunts and moans during the treatment! When he came back, he looked a lot calmer. I can only assume that he had given someone the third degree for being home with the dog, a little rich when he had been having a massage the whole time!

Anyway, he seemed pretty pleased with himself and offered me a tip – I'm not sure if it was for the massage or for grassing on whoever had the dog! He only had American dollars in cash on him which I said was fine as my partner travels a lot so it would get used.

I think he gave me around $20 which I ended up keeping until nearly a year later when I took a holiday in Washington and bought myself a souvenir with my conference call tip!

I Am Not a Masseur

Working as a mobile therapist is always a tough gig. You have a lot less control over situations such as last-minute cancellations, who your client actually is, how much space you will have to set up in, how many flights of stairs you're going to be expected to drag your massage couch up, where you're going to park and plenty of other stupid things like that.

I worked mobile for quite a few years and it was hard going. I was getting very disillusioned with the problems that you sometimes have to deal with and needed to make a change. I could tell you so many stories, some funny, some a bit scary and some just plain annoying. Like the time that I arrived at a client's house and his wife answered the door and told me to leave and that I must have the wrong address. When I called him, he apologised and said that he would not be able to have treatments any more and offered no further explanation, nor did he offer to pay any cancellation fee or reimburse me for the fuel it cost to get to his address. I can only assume that his wife had no idea that he was having treatments from me and was not happy to find out, God knows why! Or the time that I arrived at a client's house to treat a female student suffering from shoulder pain due to posture, only to find that she wanted me to massage her in her living room with four of her male housemates sat watching, and she wanted to be naked and had "turned the central heating up so there was no need for a towel." Then, of course, there is the classic question, "What 'extras' do you offer?" Funny that a foot scrub or face cleanse is never what they are hoping you will say. Or one of my favourite conversations…

CLIENT: What do you wear during a massage?

ME: If it's for a full body massage, then you just keep your underwear on and take everything else off, including jewellery.

CLIENT: That's not what I mean.

ME: Are you just looking for a back massage, because then you can keep your trousers on if you'd prefer?

CLIENT: You know what I mean.

ME: (thinking *well clearly I don't jackass or this conversation would already be over*) I am not sure what you mean, sir. Could you please explain?

CLIENT: What will you be wearing?

ME: A massage therapy tunic and a pair of trousers. That is my work uniform.

CLIENT: You won't be wearing…less?

Some of the ideas that people have about massage therapy are just way off!

To try and eliminate some of the more moronic and, frankly, insulting situations that mobile massage therapy seemed to throw up, I decided to try and find somewhere to rent and have clients visit me instead of me visiting them. For a while, I rented a room in my local town. I shared it with another therapist; she had the room five days a week and I rented it two days a week. This was meant to give me a little more stability and safety and for a short while, it was very useful. Unfortunately, it was not to last and when the other therapist decided to move on, I was given the option to either take on her days as well as just my two, something that I could not afford to do, or to leave as well. So, I was back to just mobile work while I looked for another, more affordable place. Shortly after this happened, the owners of the property decided to sell up and all the other therapists moved premises. A few months later, I was walking past the building and I noticed that a new sign had gone up saying Thai Massage Parlour. I thought nothing more of it until the phone calls started.

Now, I don't know too much about technology, I am a massage therapist not an IT technician or web designer, and I do not pretend to know a thing about how the internet works, but I have taken the time to Google my own business and I'm surprised and confused by the number of places that my business is listed. Often incorrectly! I'm not sure why this happens but it would seem that there are plenty of websites that list local massage therapists and their business details, information that I guess they must source from other online directories or maybe from Facebook, hell I don't know. All I know is that, at some point in history, a few business directories had got hold of my business details while I had been working at that treatment room address and someone, somewhere had not realised that I had ceased working from that location. I found more than ten online business listings with my name, photograph and mobile phone number, with the Thai Massage Parlour name and address. I am not one hundred per cent sure what this Thai Massage Parlour offered its customers, but from the phone calls I was getting, it was not massage therapy!

The calls started one night at around 11:30pm. I still don't know why I answered. I think when you are self-employed and young, you think that you have to answer every call, every email, every text, immediately or you might lose that business. You have this crazy notion that your time is not yours any more and that you have to be at your clients' every beck and call 24/7, weekends don't exist and your working hours never seem to end. As I have got older, and possibly as a result of this experience, I have learned that calls etc get answered during business hours only, and if anyone gets pushy or upset about that, then they are not your ideal customer and can go swivel!

So, it's 11:30pm (I don't remember what day of the week) and my phone starts ringing from a withheld or unknown number. I also now have a rule that I never answer a call if the number is missing! I pick it up and a male voice says, "Is this [uses my name]? Are you a massage therapist?"

I answer yes, feeling slightly annoyed that someone is calling me about work at such a late hour.

"I've been a bad boy and I need to be punished."

You know those moments, when it's late and you're tired and you mishear things on the phone? Well, I paused for a second, really confused, and then said, "I'm sorry, could you repeat that?"

"I'm such a baaaaaaad boy…" I hung up the phone.

A few days later, late at night, my phone rings, male voice: "Hello, is this [uses my name]?"

"Yes, it is. Can I help you?"

"I'm looking for a massage…a really deep, hard massage."

"I'm sorry, it's very late, if you need an appointment, please call during working hours to make a booking." The phone hangs up.

Another night, the phone rings late. Why I keep picking up I do not know. Male voice, breathing heavily, "Hi, is this [uses my name]?"

"No," I say, and hang the phone up.

*

54

These calls kept coming through, again and again. Getting more frequent. And, stupidly, I kept answering them. At this point, I had not Googled my business and was not aware that I was being listed as a Thai massage parlour but the phone call that made me Google myself and find out happened at about 2am one day. Groggily, I pick up the phone and say, "Hello?"

"Hi, is this [uses my full name]?" That got my attention and I started to wake up enough to not immediately slam the phone down on the heavy breathing, deep male voice.

"Yes, how can I help?"

"I need a masseuse." I HATE that word!

Bristling, I reply, "I am not a masseuse. I am a licensed massage therapist."

He pauses for a moment, "What else do you offer?"

"Nothing, I am a massage therapist and I offer professional massage."

"Oh, sorry to bother you," he said, and hung up.

I sat up in bed, completely awake and quite confused. That was the most polite, indecent phone call I had ever received. I was so angry but at the same time the guy seemed genuinely apologetic and possibly embarrassed. I couldn't get back to sleep and so I got up and ended up Googling my business. And there you have it, I found all the listings, incorrectly attaching my name and photo to a Thai massage parlour with very late opening hours. It took me a while to correct the listings, some of which I was never able to change.

Not long after that, the Thai massage parlour was closed down, rumour has it, by the police. It popped up again months later in another location but was closed down again and carried on bouncing around different locations for a while.

I did have a client visit me once who had been there for a massage. When he booked his massage, he asked if I was associated with the place and I vehemently denied this. He sounded very relieved and said that he wasn't sure if he would have booked if I had been working there. When he came for his massage, I decided to ask him about it. He told me that he had been there for a massage and was made to feel very uncomfortable. The therapist was very insistent that he take all of his clothes off, but he refused and while he was lying face down on the massage couch, the therapist started massaging his back, but then another therapist came in and started massaging his legs. He was also asked if he wanted extra.

Sometimes, it's no wonder that massage therapy gets a bad name or that everyone in the industry gets so outraged at being referred to as masseurs working from 'parlours'.

Expired

Christmas time was always a bit of a quiet period for me, and as a self-employed massage therapist with no other income, that could be super scary. Every year was the same; I would have a nice, fairly steady flow of clients throughout the year and then towards the end of November it would start to quieten down. The first week or two of December would get quieter and quieter, there would be more last-minute cancellations as people started to get into the Christmas spirit and out of their usual routine. Then the third week of December almost everyone would cancel because they still had Christmas shopping to get done or they were getting busy with parties and family etc., then Christmas week you would be completely dead, no work whatsoever, and that was terrifying! That would sometimes last well into January, people would have spent way too much over Christmas and would be struggling to find the money for self-care and I would not get back on track until the end of January, beginning of February.

When you are self-employed, it is hard to deal with these quiet periods, especially when the reason that you are quiet is because of people cancelling, rather than because you are not getting any bookings. You cannot plan anything because you have a client booked in and when they cancel, it is devastating – you lose your day's income! When you don't work, you don't get paid, and it can be so stressful. I hated the Christmas period.

One year, I had cancellation after cancellation, and even a few clients that just didn't bother turning up at all! I was desperate, so I decided that I would spend a little money on getting some nice vouchers printed out for Christmas and sell them as a lovely gift idea and get some money coming in that way. I had not done vouchers before because I was worried about fair expiry dates, maybe someone wanting a refund, or what happened when everyone wants their voucher treatment in the same month and I can't see my regular clients because I'm fully booked with vouchers and I'm then not earning what I should be that month. Maybe I worry too much or overthink things, but friends of mine who are also therapists had done vouchers and had problems, so I wanted to be sure I didn't make the same mistakes that they did.

I had my vouchers made and I sold a few before Christmas. It certainly didn't make me enough money to warrant having that time off, but it was better than nothing and took some of the stress out of Christmas for me. I made sure that each voucher had a clearly displayed expiry date, six months after the purchase date; I felt that this was more than enough time for the recipient to book a treatment in. Unbelievably, on Boxing Day my phone went off a few times with the same message, *I have been given a voucher for a massage for Christmas and I need to get a treatment booked in, when are you available?* Over the following days, between Christmas and New Year, I had a few more very similar messages.

I thought, yes, this is working, what a great idea! I was getting bookings during my normally quiet time and, although they were for vouchers and I wasn't getting paid (because I already had been paid), I was working and getting more than half of the vouchers redeemed before work picked back up again.

I was a little nervous in February, knowing that I still had a few vouchers out there that needed redeeming and having my diary filling up fast with my regular clients, but a few trickled through and I managed to fit them in, a few more in March and by April I had lost track and forgotten how many vouchers were left. I found out, or at least partially found out, in June. I started receiving a few messages, such as *hi, I have a voucher that is expiring soon and I need to book it in.* Luckily there weren't too many and I managed to get most booked in but there were a couple that left it right up until the day before the voucher expired and got shitty with me because I couldn't magically fit them in exactly when they wanted. I did the right thing, though, and replied *I'm sorry I am unable to fit you in before your voucher expires. On this occasion I will honour the voucher as long as you make your booking today and your appointment is before the end of this month.* This was fine and I got the vouchers booked in.

Mostly it went fine, and I even got a few repeat bookings who turned into regular clients, but one was very difficult. I had already agreed to honour their expired voucher but the day before their appointment they called to reschedule. I had it written in my diary that they were using an expired voucher, but I reluctantly agreed to reschedule *providing that the appointment is before the end of this month.* They rebooked for the following week which was the day before the end of the month and they never showed up! A week later they called me, "Hi, I had an appointment booked for last week but I wasn't able to attend. Can I reschedule for next week?"

"Yes, I have an available appointment but I'm afraid you will not be able to use your voucher as the voucher has expired and you missed your appointment."

"But you said you would accept my voucher."

"I would have if you had come to your appointment as planned. I have a cancellation policy and you did not let me know you were not coming."

"My kid was sick, what was I supposed to do? I need to use my voucher, it was a gift, I didn't know it expired."

"I'm sorry to hear that, but unfortunately your voucher has expired. The expiry date is written on the front and is no longer valid," and of course you know it had expired, we discussed it twice!

"You heartless bitch!" she screamed, and hung up the phone.

I was quite upset by this and decided that the following Christmas I wasn't going to put myself through the hassle of vouchers. I made my cancellation policy a bit more rigid and actually enforced it for once! I also started selling skincare products so that when the quiet period inevitably came, I still had product sales to fall back on. At Christmas they brought out beautiful Christmas gift sets which were really popular and kept the money coming in when things usually got quiet.

A while later, I had a call about a voucher. "I found a voucher, I must have been given it as a Christmas gift." Oh here we go again. "It expired a while ago, can I still use it?"

"I'm really sorry, but no. I'm afraid if it has expired a while ago, then you can't use it."

"But I have been really ill and now I want to use it. It only just expired."

"I'm sorry but I haven't offered vouchers now for over a year so the expiry will have been almost a year ago."

"It's not a year, it's less than that, and I have been ill."

"I'm sorry but no, that voucher cannot be redeemed."

I thought that was the end of that but the voucher issues just kept coming and people get so angry when you say no to them.

*

I had a new client come to see me for a treatment. When she arrived, she said, "I want to collect my free product. I have a voucher." I was completely thrown by her request; I have never given out free products.

"I'm sorry, I'm not giving out vouchers for free products."

"Oh, you didn't give it to me, it was in *The Telegraph* magazine." She handed me the voucher. It was for the same brand of products that I was selling but nothing to do with me. I had a quick scan through the small print.

"Oh, if you see here, it's only for John Lewis sites. If you go there, there's one in town, they should be able to help you."

"But I don't want to go there."

By this point I should have started her treatment and we were eating into her treatment time. "You sell these products; you should give me this free gift."

"I'm so sorry, but I'm not part of this promotion. I don't even have this product to give you. I don't stock it."

"But I want it," she demanded.

"I'm really sorry, but I can't help you. It would be like if you have a voucher to get a tin of free baked beans from one supermarket but you try to redeem it at another supermarket chain, they won't be able to do that."

"It's nothing like that. You have the same products."

"I'm sorry, but I don't even have the product that you want."

"Well, you shouldn't advertise the products if you don't have them!"

"I do have the products but I don't have that product and unfortunately I can't accept that voucher."

By this point she was missing a good chunk of her massage and I hadn't even got her in the treatment room yet!

"This is ridiculous. I don't have to listen to this. You shouldn't be allowed to advertise those products. I should speak to your manager."

"I'm self-employed. I don't have a manager."

At that, she turned around in a huge huff and disappeared without having her treatment, or her free product that I didn't even have!

I didn't bother trying to implement my cancellation policy. I didn't think I would get anywhere with that.

Part Three

Let's Hear It for the Boys

I overheard two of my clients talking about me in the relaxation room of the spa I was working in. One was graphically describing my body when the other turned to her and said, "Oh I know, the things I would do to him, it's such a waste that he's gay." Without thinking, I loudly said, "Oh dear, my wife will be upset!" and walked out.

Very occasionally when a guy gets really relaxed and sleeps during a massage, it can result in them getting an erection. It's nothing to be embarrassed about, it's a normal bodily function, just the same as people fart when they get relaxed, but so many guys get mortified when that happens with me and start yelling, "I swear I'm not gay, mate." Nothing makes a guy act more butch than that!

Go Deeper

I'm not going to lie, I was a young man when I got into massage therapy, a boy really, and I one hundred per cent did it for the women. I was turning twenty, awkward and horny. My massage instructor was an old soul and a registered GP who had given up his practice to focus on the holistic side of medical care and teach the importance of the mind, body energy link. He saw right through me straight away.

I have a huge amount of respect for how that man taught me. The anatomy knowledge that he bestowed upon me very early on, and continued to build upon throughout my training, kicked any filthy thoughts straight out of my head. Within weeks, if I had a beautiful woman lying naked on the couch before me, all I could see were muscles, tendons, attachments, pressure points, lymphatics, nervous systems – a complex and incredible organic machine.

I thought I would find an easy way to get closer to a lot of women, and instead I found a fascinating career that I still cherish and have a huge amount of respect for. I love this industry; even though I have changed industries many times, I am still followed by and drawn back to holistic therapies.

One of my first jobs was based within a block of flats in a capital city housing mostly celebrities, models and the higher class of society. It was a fairly daunting place to go to for work as a newly qualified, young massage therapist.

One of my clients was a stunning, slender, female model. The first time I visited her, she made it very clear that she needed a deep massage treatment. She was quite demanding and adamant that she'd had many massages before and needed to have a very deep, hard massage. Her frame, however, was incredibly slim and I was not convinced that the treatment she was demanding was actually suitable for her. I tried to explain to her that the style of massage therapy that I offered, although firm, was not a deep tissue style and was more holistic; this did not change her mind and she continued with her demands. I then went on to explain why, in my professional opinion, a deep massage would just cause pain, and possibly more damage than good, to her muscle tissue and I did not think that it was wise to be using my full strength on her body. She agreed, got on the couch and I began her treatment.

Starting my treatment through the towel, I could feel that there was a lot of tension, especially in her back and upper shoulders. Before I could even start the actual treatment, she was already demanding a deeper pressure. Once again, explaining that I needed to first warm up her muscle tissue to avoid damage, I continued with my treatment but started with a few pressure points to both loosen muscles but also to show her that a deeper treatment would be more painful than relaxing. Holding the pressure points in the tops of her shoulders, close to her neck, I expected the inevitable discomfort and then release of tension to satisfy her demands, but it did not.

Pulling the towel back to begin the massage, I uncovered the whole of her back and the top of her buttocks and began to apply oil and warm her muscles. She started to moan softly as I treated her, making me believe that she would finally accept the treatment that she needed. Pretty soon she started asking for a deeper massage. I gradually increased my pressure to where I thought I could safely treat but I refused to go any firmer for fear of causing more damage. She continued to occasionally groan or mumble, and then shouted, "Go deeper."

It was then that the door slid open and a six-foot tall, balding man, glared into the room at me. I can only assume this was her husband, he was never introduced. He continued staring at me for a few minutes while I did my best to ignore his glares and continue with my work, and my client continued to moan. I have no idea how long he was there for. I zoned him, and the groaning, out and continued with my work. He was nowhere to be seen when I left.

A week or so later, I was booked again by the same woman, and as before, she insisted that she needed a deep, hard massage and I insisted that it would be more damaging than beneficial for her to have the level of pressure that she was demanding. Once again, she agreed with me and we started the session. Exactly the same as before, she started moaning and, as before, I just got into my own rhythm and flow and did my best to block out her noises.

Working on her lower back elicited a similar reaction to the last time and she started shouting, "Go deeper, harder, harder…" The same door slid open, only this time to reveal a different man. This one was enormous, he looked more like a bouncer at a nightclub, completely bald, arms so big he looked like he could kill a man with one punch. He threw the door all the way open, stepped into the room and folded his meaty arms across his chest. He never said a word, just stood there and stared. His presence made it significantly more difficult to ignore the awkwardness, but my client seemed not to notice at all and spent the rest of the treatment alternatively moaning and shouting, "Go deeper," while he angrily looked on.

Performing a full body massage to a moaning client with her husband/boyfriend/lover, or whoever he was, watching over me like a very angry hawk was probably the most challenging moment of my massage career.

Needless to say, when she contacted me again to confirm her next treatment, I had to politely decline.

A Shocking Piece of Work

I quite enjoy a couples' treatment. I know that there are many therapists who don't, but I love them. I find it nice to work with someone else. We spend the majority of our working life in silence while our customers snooze their treatment time away, then in between clients, we are just too busy to have a chat or catch up with a conscious human being, so the couples' treatments are the only time you get to really interact with someone. True, this all has to be done in mime and with exaggerated facial expressions, but that's half of the fun! The day certainly goes by a lot quicker when you get to do the odd couples' treatment.

We had had a few couples' bookings that day and luckily it had been properly planned out so that I had been working with the same therapist all day. We had got into a really good rhythm with consultations, timings of the treatments and turning the room around quickly. The day was going brilliantly and we were almost done, just one more couples' full body massage and we were finished for the day.

Our clients were seated in the waiting room, filling out their consultation forms. Our receptionist came up to the room to let us know that they had arrived and that they were on a wedding package with the hotel. They were getting married at the hotel, so there were a few extra special touches that we needed to make sure we were covering, such as making sure we had a glass of champagne waiting for them when their treatment ended.

We collected the clients from the waiting room and took them up the stairs to the couples' room. We had the obligatory small talk exchange as we went and found out that they were getting married in just two days' time. We left the pair to get ready and get on the massage couches. When we went back into the room to start the treatments, the groom-to-be was lying on my massage bed and the bride-to-be was on the other therapist's bed.

We started the treatments with our usual welcome rituals and pressure points, working beautifully in sync with each other. We reached the top of the couch and pressed down on the shoulders at exactly the same time, perfect rhythms! We both pulled the towels down to uncover the backs of our clients and, you know when someone has had a homemade tattoo? Well, all that was written on my client's back was *Magaluf Fuckin' Mental 2013*, in a scrawling, uneven, (what looked like a child's handwriting) horrific mess! It was quite small, but even so, I couldn't help but think, why would anyone want to marry someone with *Magaluf Fuckin' Mental 2013* scrawled on their back? For me, that would be a deal breaker!

I must have taken a little longer trying to read this spider print and the other therapist had already started massaging the bride. She looked up at me to see what had stopped me, and as I started the treatment, I was nodding my head at her and pointedly looking down at this awful tattoo. As she came around the couch to work on the other side of her client's back, she had a look over at the tattoo and mouthed, "*What the fuck?!*" pulling a disgusted face.

At the end of the treatment, we went out of the room to allow the couple to get ready. The other therapist looked at me and said, "Why would you do that to yourself?"

"I would demand for that to be removed before I agreed to get married to him!" I replied.

"At the very least, he could have it covered with something less shit."

We went and got the champagne ready for the couple and took them through to the relaxation room. At least the whole thing sparked an interesting conversation about the worst tattoos that we had ever seen during a massage treatment. Of course, you have the ones that are spelled wrong or the ones that are clearly chosen during a drunken moment or the ones that are just drawn really badly (usually faces). As a massage therapist, tattoos are actually quite nice because you get something to look at or read during a massage, and it just breaks the routine up a bit in a long day!

This conversation led me to telling the other therapist about the worst tattoo I had ever seen, which was during a massage once when I worked in a spa in Australia.

I was working in a really nice posh, fancy spa. It was one of the highest rated spas in Australia at that time and it was based in a beautiful tower block hotel, right on the river bank in Melbourne. It had loads of dual treatment rooms for couples' treatments. They had a two-and-a-half-hour package which included a Geisha tub with nibbles, smoothies etc. and then a facial and hot stones massage. Generally, the couples would spend around half an hour in the tub and then you would have forty-five minutes to one hour for the facial and then an hour or hour and fifteen minutes for the full body hot stones massage. As you were going from facial to massage, you would start the massage on the chest and arms, moving down to the fronts of the legs and feet and then turn your client over to start on the backs of the legs and finish with a long back, neck and shoulder massage. It was a really lovely, indulgent treatment, and very popular (and expensive)!

A gay couple had booked the treatment with me and my colleague, who happened to be a male therapist. As usual with a couples' treatment, the therapist picks which bed they prefer to work on, and whichever client is on that bed, that is the client that you will be working on. We let the clients know that it was time for them to get out of the Geisha tub and get themselves ready on the massage beds for their facials and we left the room for them to get ready. When we came back into the room, the client on my couch was the more slender of the two, and his partner, who was a bigger, more muscular build, was on the male therapist's couch. I mean, in all honesty, if you could come up with the two worst stereotypes for gay men, they were in the relationship together – the slender one was very effeminate and the other, very butch. They were a really lovely couple and so nice, so we were looking forward to doing their treatments. It always makes the treatment more relaxing when the couple's energy is nice.

We started the facials, and everything was really relaxed and quiet. The music was playing softly in the background, the lights were turned down low but were still bright enough to see what you were doing so you could select the right products for each client's skin type and the clients were both quiet and relaxed. The other therapist put the hot stones heaters on while we had the facial masks on and we used the time to prepare for the next stage of the treatment and to perform a lovely scalp massage. I always get a bit sleepy doing scalp massages, I find them so relaxing to do.

So, we are all totally blissed out as we finish the facials and start with the hot stones. All goes really smoothly and we both finish at the same time on the client's feet. We go back up to the top of the couches and whisper to our clients, at the same time, that it is time to roll over. As always, we carefully lifted the towels from the opposite side of the couch to where we were standing, so we did not see any of the client's body as they turned over.

Then, with the clients lying face down, we started the back of body massage, from the ankles up.

I noticed that my client had a tattoo on his back and when I finally got to that part of the massage, I pulled back the towel to reveal a giant tattoo of a hummingbird. It was so detailed, fully coloured and almost jumped out of his skin. Absolutely beautiful.

Still feeling totally blissed out with this treatment, I was just going with the flow and letting the hot stones do their thing. The low light, soft music and relaxed ambience make these the best treatments to do and I felt totally connected with my work and my mind was just drifting off. A long treatment like this can almost be a meditation for the therapist and I was completely unaware of my colleague's discomfort until he accidentally let out a strange, low, almost whimpering sound.

He was also working on his client's back, who also had a giant tattoo, very detailed and realistic, probably done by the exact same tattoo artist. This tattoo was a full back piece, on a very muscular, very broad, large man, so it was a big tattoo and, did I mention already, very, very detailed.

The reason for the male therapist's discomfort was the nature of the tattoo. It was a karma sutra type picture of two men wrapped around each other and it looked so real. Just like the hummingbird on my client, this tattoo really jumped out of his skin at you. One of the men in the tattoo had a whacking great big cock, and the other man had the end of it in his mouth. The poor therapist was having to perform long sweeping effleurage movements up and down a picture of an erect penis and just to add insult to injury, the client seemed to have a lot of muscular tension, halfway up the shaft.

I couldn't stop looking over at the other client. My flow was shot and I was trying desperately not to make any noise. The male therapist was trying desperately not to look at the penis, which was effectively in his hands, and trying to continue the massage quietly and professionally. We were both very shocked and the poor male therapist was desperate to finish the treatment but unfortunately, because the massage routine started on the front of the body and ended with the back massage, we still had another half an hour to go and only the back left to treat.

My poor colleague had to stroke a dick pic for half an hour! That's a day he is unlikely to forget in a hurry.

Part Four

It Happens to the Best of Us (When Therapists Get It Wrong)

My first ever job as a mobile massage therapist was at a hotel. I was so nervous, I arrived early with my massage couch and enough towels for a rugby team. However, when I went to the guest room and started to get set up, I realised I had no oil with me! I had to steal the complementary bottle of body lotion from the bathroom. If that wasn't bad enough, he enjoyed his massage so much that he asked if I could stay and do a full body massage instead of just back, neck and shoulders. I had run out of lotion, so I had to fake another booking!

Trying to hold in a sneeze when you are in the middle of a massage! It's so hard but I have now perfected the inward sneeze. It took a while though. I once tried to hold back a sneeze but it went horribly wrong and I ended up making the weirdest, loudest sound in the middle of a relaxing massage.

When you're working in a spa and your client has filled out their consultation form but their handwriting is appalling and you cannot figure out what their name is, so you have to just walk up to random guests and introduce yourself, hoping that eventually you will find the right person and they will tell you their name – and then they still don't tell you their name.

A Fanny Feeling

A lot of the stories in this book are about clients that have been behaving inappropriately or are maybe a bit clueless, classless, confused or awkward, so I thought it would be a bit of a change to share a story, not of a client behaving badly, but of a therapist, perhaps making a bit of a judgement error...

This story is from when I was working at a big spa in the south of the UK with ten treatment rooms over two floors. It was a very busy and popular spa with the dreaded five-minute turnaround time! For those of you lucky enough to not know what that means, a five-minute turnaround is the time that you have from the moment that you finish your treatment to the moment that you collect your next guest from reception. It is an absolute killer! You have got to wait for your client to get dressed, take them to the relaxation room, give them aftercare advice and a glass of water, get back to your room, clean up, change towels, prepare for your next treatment and collect your next guest, all in five minutes!

All without looking like you are rushing! It is an impossible task which every therapist hates, and makes the job more of a cattle market than a therapeutic, relaxation experience. And with it being a busy spa, you are most likely going to get a thirty-minute break in an eight-and-a-half-hour day and be back-to-back with clients from start to finish. Catching up, cleaning up, having a toilet break are all luxuries that, in a busy day, you are just not going to get. So, with that in mind, sometimes you have to run for a wee while your client is changing, or you're going to be doing the cross-legged wee dance through the whole of your next treatment!

We were using DECLEOR products in the spa at that time. I love DECLEOR, they use aromatherapy products for every treatment; even in a massage, you are encouraged to start and finish your treatments with suitable aromatherapy products.

This treatment was a full body deep tissue massage, so you would massage each area of the body and then use the CIRCULAGEL reviving toning gel to work into the muscles to finish each section. CIRCULAGEL is an arnica-based product designed to relieve tired, aching muscles, improve circulation and energise and firm muscles. From that brief description, you can probably guess that it leaves the skin feeling quite tingling, a bit like using a strong mint essential oil.

I was doing this full body massage on a really busy day. Straight after this massage, I had another twenty-five-minute treatment before my lunch break and then another four or so hours left of my shift. I was booked up all day with no break other than my lunch break. Luckily, the room that I was in was across the corridor from the only toilet on that floor, so I would be able to dash in and out while my client was changing if I needed to (and, of course, if it was free). The massage went absolutely fine and I finished the last part of the massage and applied the final CIRCULAGEL. The sink in my room was properly tiny! I washed my hands as best and as quietly as I could, but I must have still had the gel on my hands and wrists as I left the room and rushed across to the toilet for a quick wee while my client was getting ready. I totally didn't think about the gel.

I had to be super quick because my client was just getting back into a robe and wouldn't take long to get dressed. I had a wee and I was completely fine, pulled my trousers up and washed my hands, then ran back out to wait for my client. But that is when things started to go very badly wrong! Just as my client was coming out of the room, my moo-moo literally caught on fire!

I had to take them downstairs to the relaxation room, get them a glass of water and do my best to smile and pretend that everything was fine, and then I hurried back up to get ready for the next client. I was almost limping coming back up the stairs! My fanny was burning so bad!

Another therapist was coming back from the relaxation room and I told her what I had done. She laughed but didn't react like this was that shocking, so maybe it has happened to someone else before, but she said, "Why don't you use one of the wet wipes for the Hollywood waxing to get it off?"

Funnily enough, adding water to CIRCULAGEL does not make it any better!

You hear people saying that that minty shower gel is bad for your moo moo but this is something else! It was horrific! The wipes made it so much worse but I had no choice but to go straight back to the reception to collect my next client! I honestly don't know how I managed to keep going through my next treatment, I couldn't tell you anything about it and I just thank God it was only one treatment before lunch! I had to plaster that classic therapist smile on my face and keep repeating to myself, "I'm fine, everything's fine!" whilst inside I was screaming while my moo carried on burning!

I don't know how long it took for the effects of that to wear off, but I swear I will never, ever do that again! Now, if I ever have to touch CIRCULAGEL, I scrub my hands to death before I do anything else!

You're Feeling Very Sleepy!

One of the things that bothered me most about working in a spa were the lights, or lack thereof. I spent just over a year working in a spa where all of the treatment rooms were windowless and the dimmer switches didn't dim enough. You had a choice of either lights on or lights off! Everyone knows that part of the massage experience is how the room itself is set up. Most massage treatment rooms have very soft, low lighting and are designed to look warm, cosy and safe. The idea behind treatment room design is that you want to mimic the womb; that safety and security of pre-birth. Even the music, especially whale music, is meant to give the comfort and feeling of being back in your mother's womb. And so it is that most treatment rooms are dark or very dimly lit while the treatment is taking place. However, in this spa the choice was clear: have the lights blaring right into the client's eyes (if they are lying face up on the couch), or have them turned off and hope you don't fall over anything.

The management in this spa were all for dim lights but did nothing to provide this. They made no investment in lamps or just getting the dimmer switches fixed or changed. They did, however, provide us with tealight candles, but these were limited due to the 'expense'!

I think my eyes might have suffered permanently from my year of working in the near darkness! We would have four or five tealight candles per room per day and on an eight-hour shift, the candles would not last the whole day through, so you had to be careful when you used them and how many you used at a time. For facial treatments, you definitely needed all the candles, although there were plenty of times that I didn't have enough light and I wouldn't know until they walked out of the room that I had left mask or other products on my client's nose or throat. For massage, I tended to close my eyes during treatments, perhaps as a result of candlelit working, I'm not sure, but I could get away with just one tealight if I had to. For Indian head massage, too, you could do with just one.

There were plenty of times that you would be part way through a treatment, usually towards the end of the day, and all your candles would just burn out and you were plunged into complete darkness. The only other light in the room was the tiny green indicator light on the smoke alarm to let you know it was working, but this didn't illuminate anything.

In a rare effort to try and make our working lives a little easier, management bought in slightly larger tealights for a short while. They did burn for a little longer than the regular ones but didn't give off any extra light.

It was towards the end of a long, massage filled day and I was pretty exhausted. I had one client left and, thank goodness, it was an Indian head massage instead of a back massage. I was overjoyed at the thought of being able to sit down and take the weight off my poor feet for the next twenty-five minutes. I went to collect my client from reception and the receptionist urgently beckoned me over to her. We went into the small office behind her desk and she whispered to me, "Oh my God, you're so lucky! Your client is beautiful!"

Checking the consultation form, I confirmed that my client was a man in his early thirties.

"He's just in the changing rooms, he is soooo fit!" the receptionist carried on.

I was too tired to be in any way excited, and besides, her taste in men did not match my own at all. I heard the reception door open and waited for the receptionist to look out to see who it was.

"Oh God, he's here. You're so lucky!" she exclaimed again.

I walked out of the little office to greet my client. I was still scanning through the consultation form and hadn't really looked at him. I extended my hand and introduced myself and looked up just as he replied.

I have no idea what he said! I really hope my mouth wasn't hanging open, but it could have been. WOW!

Sat in front of me in a white, short(ish) robe was the most beautiful man I had ever seen. He was like a young Lenny Kravitz. When he stood up, I think I audibly gulped! He was definitely over six-feet tall, slender, black skin, afro hair and absolutely stunning. I made some lame comment about him being too tall for the massage couch as I took him through to the candlelit treatment room for his Indian head massage.

I explained the treatment to him and left the room for him to get ready. Standing outside the treatment room, I mouthed, "*Oh my God*," to the receptionist and she mouthed back, "*I know!*"

Heading back into the treatment room, I moved my little salon stool to the head of the couch and sat down to start the treatment. The music was soft and soothing, the aromatherapy oils I was using were lavender based and relaxing. The candle gently flickered in the corner to my right and the rest of the room was dark. My client relaxed almost immediately. The only sounds he made were his soft exhales of breath.

I allowed myself to get lost in the music and the gentle flow of my massage. It was so nice to be able to sit down after such a long day. I was absolutely exhausted, and I could feel my eyelids drooping.

I don't know if the grunt/snore came from the client or from me! My eyes snapped open and I suddenly realised that my face was inches away from his and I had been fast asleep! I had no idea what time it was and if I had snored or not! My spine snapped up straight and I did my best to continue the massage one-handed whilst searching for the time. My fob watch (like nurses have) was pinned to the waist of my trousers and I struggled to see the hands in the dark room. My eyes must have managed to adjust after having been closed for goodness knows how long because the hands of the clock came into view and I could tell that I still had ten minutes to go. Thank God, I must have nodded off and not been asleep!

I raised my head back up and continued massaging with both hands. It seemed so much lighter in the room now.

The candle in the corner was not flickering in the corner of my eye any more. Feeling a gentle sense of alarm creeping up my spine, I turned to my right to look properly at the tealight. It was definitely not flickering any more; it was far more violent than that! The sides of the tealight had caught on fire and the flame was now reaching so high that it was singeing the bottom of the shelf, nearly two foot above it! There were rolled towels and a box of paper pants on the shelf with the candle and it looked like they could go up at any time. I could actually feel the heat from the flame against my cheek. I was still massaging!

Without skipping a beat, I continued my massage, again one-handed. I reached down to my left where I had a plastic cup with a little water left in it. Skilfully swapping hands, I passed the cup into my right hand and turned my stool towards the angry candle. My heart was in my throat as I simultaneously massaged my client's head and reached towards on open flame. Quickly and carefully, I tipped the cup and its content over on the candle and left the cup over the tealight to stop any oxygen getting into it and relighting it. The room was instantly plunged into complete darkness and I carried on with the final few minutes of my treatment.

I finished the treatment, let my client know that his treatment had come to an end and asked him if he was ready for me to put the lights up or if he would rather I left them off. He said to leave them off, and I left the room to wait for him to get ready and leave.

The receptionist had already gone home for the day so there was no one there for me to tell what had happened with the candle, so I wrote a note. I didn't mention that I had nearly fallen asleep on my client's face though.

When he came out of the room, he thanked me for the treatment and didn't mention anything about me falling asleep or a potential fire hazard, so I assumed that he had slept through it all. He left the spa, and I went back into the treatment room to clear up and assess the damage.

The plastic cup had started to melt from the heat but the flame was out. There was a little water on the shelf and the floor but not much. The candle was still too hot to touch and even after it cooled down, it was stuck fast to the shelf. The white, rolled up towels were a little black but hopefully washable and the shelf above had a huge scorch mark and was hot to the touch.

I cleaned up as best as I could.

The spa continued to use the large tealight candles, even after a couple of the other therapists had similar experiences. I don't think they bought any more though.

To this day, I am a little bit scared of the big tealights!

Getting Up

Naivety doesn't last long in this business. I was very young and very naïve when I first started my massage practice. That changed very quickly. I must have been around nineteen when this particular story happened.

I had not been working as a massage therapist for very long; I would have finished my first massage qualification earlier that same year and was still in training but able to get my insurance for massage to start working straight away. Only having a qualification in massage and not yet anything else meant that I was struggling to find work and so had to set up as self-employed for the time being, working out of my living room.

I was a member with a large directory of complementary therapists through my insurance, and at that time, they had a register for their members with all of their qualifications and contact details. I honestly cannot remember if I was trained in aromatherapy at this point or if I was still studying for it or just waiting for the certificate, but I do remember that a client got in touch with me, via the directory, wanting an aromatherapy massage.

I had never had a client outside of my social circle before and I was both nervous and excited that someone had found my details and chosen to have a treatment with me through the directory's website. There were so many other therapists who were better established, more qualified and more experienced than me. I was a bit overwhelmed by it all and found myself babbling nervously on the phone to him about his booking. I must have given him the directions to the house three or four times over the phone and then again via text message.

When he arrived, I made sure I did everything exactly by the book and exactly how my teachers had told me. I had made sure I had a coat stand by the door for him and a seat for him to sit down on and take his shoes off before coming into the living room. I had the lengthiest consultation form ever; over the years I have seriously condensed down my consultation forms and I can't believe the amount of irrelevant data you used to have to collect for every client. I think it was close to four pages long! He very dutifully sat down and carefully went through the whole form, filling out all his personal data, including details of his children (I distinctly remember him having a daughter the same age as me), pets, hobbies, then the health questionnaire (more detailed than the ones you get from the GP), sleep patterns, stress levels etc., etc.

Then there was the second form to fill out to choose the right oils to use. I did tell you I was working by the book!

When this was finally all completed, I asked him about his reasons for treatment and his expectations and he confirmed that he wanted to have a full body, relaxing, aromatherapy massage. I then explained the treatment, told him what he needed to do next – remove jewellery, watches etc., keep underwear on but all other clothing off, including socks, and lie face down on the bed under the towel provided. I went to wash my hands in the bathroom while he got ready for his treatment.

The treatment went perfectly despite my nervousness at the beginning. I found my confidence as I worked and performed the perfect relaxing massage, I even had to wake him up to get him to turn over on the couch. My timings were perfect, I had mixed myself enough of the massage oil with the essential oils he had picked out and I was feeling super happy about the whole treatment. He had been asleep for most of it and I was a bit concerned about him getting up too quickly. My massage couch was static and the head would not raise for him to be sat up at the end of his treatment so I wanted to make sure that he was safe getting off the couch, but my training also dictated that I should leave to give him the privacy to get up on his own.

Not sure what to do for the best and not wanting to disturb his zen-like state, I softly whispered to him, "That's the end of your massage. Do you need me to help you get up?"

He gave me a very odd look and I was worried that because he had been asleep, maybe he felt that he had been cheated on the timings. "No, I think I'm OK," he replied, and I smiled with relief and said, "I will give you some privacy and go and wash my hands."

When I came back from the bathroom, he was stood next to the couch, completely naked and fully erect. He had his hands on his hips and his shoulders leaned slightly back as though he were thrusting his erect penis at me. I couldn't help but stare, my brain not quite switching on to what was happening.

He stood there staring back at me for, I have no idea how long, and I just stood there staring, not moving or saying a word, with no clue what was happening.

"Well, what now?" he said, pointing at his erect penis just in case I hadn't noticed it.

I cleared my throat and slowly said, "Now, you get dressed and you pay me for your massage and then you leave."

His shoulders visibly sank as he reached for his undies and started to awkwardly and quickly get dressed. I carried on just standing there and watched him put the cash on the table, grab his coat and leave my house.

I am not sure how many times I ran those events through my head before I realised my mistake.

I got on the phone to a friend of mine, telling her all about it, while she gasped, screamed and laughed.

At some point during that recounting it struck me: "Oh my God! I asked him if he needed help getting up?!"

She cried with laughter as I realised with horror what I had actually said and why that could have been so horrendously misinterpreted! I know exactly what I meant, which was help getting off the couch, but no wonder he gave me such a strange look! And I actually whispered that in his ear!

A few weeks later he got in contact with me, again via the directory, requesting another treatment. I declined and blocked his details so he could not contact me again.

Talk about saying the wrong thing!

Take It Off

A few years ago, I was working in a spa on a casual contract while I was continuing my studies. It's a great way to be able to keep earning whilst studying and keep your foot in the beauty industry door.

I loved my job and my work mates, even the clients we had were all really friendly and nice. You hear a lot of stories from other therapists about how awful some clients can be, but I guess I am just really lucky to have never come across that at all. That isn't to say that there have never been any challenges or slightly awkward moments, especially in beauty therapy and as a nail technician, but I guess that will have to wait for another time.

I remember this one client that I had at the spa, he came with a group of his mates, I think it might have been a stag do or something like that. They were all a little bit rowdy but well natured and they might have had a drink, but none owned up to that!

I remember my client had an unusual name that I found hard to pronounce. All the girls took their clients through to the treatment rooms first so that I didn't have to try and pronounce my client's name and get it wrong! Instead, I waited until he was the only one left and then introduced myself as his therapist and hoped that he would respond with his name, which he didn't! So, I was already feeling a little bit awkward and nervous when I took him into the treatment room. I could tell that he was really nervous too, so I did my best to explain the treatment to him and asked if there was anything I needed to know about, but he just kept nodding his head at me and I realised that he didn't speak English all that well.

I was fairly new to the spa and to spa treatments, which only added to me being nervous about not saying his name properly. I had heard so many horror stories too, so I didn't want to say the wrong thing or have any awkward moments with clients taking too much clothing off or anything like that. I tried to sort of mime what he needed to do. I carefully pulled back a bit of the top towel and said, "Lie face down," and sort of mimicked lying down on the couch, "under the towel." I lifted the top towel a bit more. He nodded a lot so I thought it was OK and I started to leave the room. He touched his shirt and said, "Take off?" I panicked a bit, not wanting him to take too much clothing off so I nodded and said, "Yes, please, take your top half off and you can leave trousers on." I pointed at my trousers. He smiled and nodded and I left the room.

I put the consultation form away and gave it a few more seconds while I tried to listen at the door. When I thought he was ready, I tapped on the door, opened it a bit and asked if I could come in. I'm not sure if he didn't understand or didn't hear me but there was no reply, so I carefully peeped through the door and stepped through.

He was lying face down on the couch with the towel covering him and I could see he had left his trousers on, which was perfect. I started to relax and took my shoes off ready to start the treatment. He was booked in for just a back massage so it seemed simpler to tell him to keep trousers on, especially because he seemed so nervous and I was worried about the language barrier.

I got my oils ready and pulled the towel back to show his back, but I noticed his shirt was still on!

I started to feel a bit frustrated, I didn't know how else to ask him to take off his t-shirt, but I then realised that he had pulled his t-shirt up and taken his arms out of the sleeves but left it around his neck. I thought maybe I could deal with it and maybe he was just so nervous that he didn't want to take his t-shirt all the way off, so I didn't say anything. I started the massage, but I was worried about getting oil on his t-shirt, so I tried to tug it up a little bit to reveal more of his back. After a little while of me struggling with the t-shirt, he lifted his head and took hold of the t-shirt and said, "Take off?"

Relieved, I said yes, and he took his t-shirt off and I carried on the massage. It was only then that I realised my mistake.

When I had said "Take your top half off", I had meant anything that he was wearing on the top half of his body needed to be taken off but he had interpreted it as take your top, half off. The poor man must have been so confused! I still feel really stupid about it!

Nice Ring

There is always that one therapist in a team that is the ditzy one, the accident prone one, the noisy one, the clumsy one, the one that will always say the wrong thing, etc. There is always one, and that one is me!

I am the therapist that drops the hot stones in the middle of a couple's massage treatment. I am the therapist that tries to glide gracefully around the couch, like all the other girls do but instead, accidentally arse-bumps the display stand and knocks over all the facial products. I am the therapist that walks up to a client and says, "Hi, I'm your therapist today. Are you ready to come through for your pregnancy massage?" only to be met with a very stern gaze and a curt, "I am not pregnant," followed by an awkward, "Oopsie, sorry, I must have the wrong details."

Arrghhh! I am the therapist who mixes the face mask with too much water and then cannot control the spread of mask into hair, ears, dribbles down the chin, blah! I am also the therapist who mixes that same mask but with not enough water and then has to attempt to spread sticky, fast setting porridge over a client's face and keep it, somehow, relaxing! I am the therapist that, when walking a couple towards the couples' treatment room asks the innocent question, "So, how long have you been together?" to be met with the very short answer, "This is my son." In my defence on that one, I think it is very odd to book a couples' treatment with your son, who looks old enough to be your boyfriend. I am THAT therapist!

I could probably write my own book with all the stories I have of silly things I have done or accidentally said at work. One of my (I think favourites is the wrong term) most memorable awkward moments was working in a spa that was based in a town house. Our prep room was on the top floor and there was a long private staircase leading from the parking at the back entrance all the way up to the prep room. We kept all of our belongings in the prep room and at the end of every shift, we would all file down the long staircase to the staff parking out the back. There were two light switches at the bottom of the staircase:one for the outside light and one for the whole of the stairs. Everyone knew that if you flipped that switch, every flight of stairs would be plunged into darkness. It was winter and so pitch black at 6:30pm when we are all trying to leave the spa for the day.

We were walking down the stairs when all of a sudden, the girl at the very bottom of the staircase flipped the wrong switch and we were all in complete and total darkness. I screamed and a few of the other girls screamed too. The girl behind me definitely screamed but that might not have been because of the darkness. In my panic, I had tried to grab for a handrail, but I had got all switched around and confused and I had accidentally reached out and grabbed the therapist behind me – in her crotch. The light came back on and I was just stood there with a fist full of fanny and the other therapist looking shocked and angry down at me! Now, I know that as therapists we have very little clue of personal space, but I think I may have taken it a little too far!

By now, you should be getting something of an idea of the kind of person that I am, so the following might come as little surprise to you. I do not think before I speak and I am easily flustered into panicked reactions that may not necessarily be socially acceptable. As this book is specifically about massage therapy, I thought I should share one final story and it should be a massage-based one.

To this day, I am amazed that I didn't get a complaint from this lady, or at the very least, lose her as one of my regular clients!

I was working in the same town house-based spa as the unfortunate crotch-grabbing incident. The spa had a really great members package and so we had a lot of local, regular customers as well as the usual holiday, special occasion or party bookings. With there being such a great return rate, the therapists often ended up being specifically requested or rebooking the same client into their diary.

I had been seeing this one lady for years, mostly for beauty treatments but also for regular massage therapy. You get really close and friendly to your regular clients and, especially with beauty treatments, you do end up gossiping a lot and learning everything there is to know about their lives. She was booked in for a full body massage with me and, although we had started off with our usual catch up and friendly chat, by the time I had finished massaging the back of her left leg and started on the right, we were both in the flow of the massage, quiet and relaxed. I finished massaging the back of her right leg and started the pressure walks up the body, laying my palms flat over her feet, walking up to her calves, backs of her thighs, a little push on her buttocks, then lower back, shoulder blades and tops of her shoulders. I pulled the towel back to uncover her back. I always work very low on her back and do a bit of work over her glutes, so I pulled the towel nice and low to reveal most of her backside and her hands. She wasn't wearing any underwear.

I got some more oil from the bottle and came back to her lower back. I pressed my palms into her lower back and slid my hands up to her shoulders, down her sides and back to her lower back. I did this three times and on my third time, I noticed that she was wearing an engagement ring that I had never seen her wear before. I had known her for long enough to know when she met her boyfriend and we had talked a lot about him and their relationship. My brain was buzzing excitedly with questions and I was losing my focus with all the excitement.

My next massage move was where I fan out from her lower back, around her hips and press into her glutes, the muscles in her bum. I was using a fair amount of pressure, so this movement did, sort of, part the cheeks a little bit. Just as I was doing that movement, my brain couldn't hold in all the excitement and I ended up blurting out, "Oh honey, you've got such a lovely ring."

There was a long pause, I thought maybe because she had been relaxing and I had disturbed her, typical me!

Eventually she said, "Um, I'm not sure how I am supposed to respond to that."

I was a bit confused and it took a little while for it to slowly dawn on me that she might have thought I had been looking at a different sort of ring. By the time I had realised what I had said, she had reached her fingertips down to the towel and was slowly shuffling the towel up to cover her crack. I just carried on with the massage, too mortified to apologise or to try and make it right.

She did not make any eye contact with me when she turned over for the front of her body to be massaged. The massage continued on, seemingly to take forever, in absolute silence (save for the quiet spa music in the background). I don't think I said anything when I finished the treatment. I might have just walked out and waited outside for her to get ready, I can't remember. I just know that I wanted to disappear! I was so embarrassed, and I can't begin to think how she must have felt.

She did make another appointment with me to get her nails done a few weeks later, so I guess it can't have been that bad! We never did speak about it.

Part Five

You Just Can't Make This S**t Up

One of my regular clients used to love having his feet massaged at the end of his treatment. One day he genuinely asked me if he could massage my feet instead. Turns out he had a foot fetish and had been fantasising about touching my feet. He is no longer a client.

When working in a spa, I always leave the room for my client to get ready, lie on the couch and cover themselves with a towel. I check they are ready before I re-enter the room. One client said that he was ready, and I walked back in to find him lying face up on the couch on top of the towel he was meant to cover himself with, completely naked with a massive boner.

Close to the Edge

Without a doubt, my most memorable client was a website enquiry I had a few years ago. I will never forget it! Not the enquiry itself, because that was pretty normal and mundane, but the actual treatment was a huge eye opener for me.

As appears to be a bit of a theme with the stories in this book, I struggle now to believe how naïve I have been at times in my career. You would think that a profession that deals with people undressing and sharing very intimate details about themselves would toughen you up a bit, open your eyes to some people's behaviour and maybe even make you more cynical about people and the world, but for so many of us, it seems to have the opposite effect. I cannot help but laugh at my complete lack of understanding whenever I recount this story.

Most of my clients initially get in touch with me via my website and this one was no exception. In fact, it was very unexceptional. He was looking to have a Hawaiian massage. I offer Lomi Lomi massages and he had had this style before and found it very relaxing. The enquiry was completely normal, there were no weird cues or vibes from the enquiry or from him when he came to see me. He was a perfectly polite guy: tall, skinny, slightly geeky (his profession was in IT and he presented as a bit of a computer geek), grey haired, about 50 or slightly above. I remember him having really long, skinny legs that slightly hung off the end of the couch, but only slightly!

When he turned up, he introduced himself politely and filled out his consultation form as normal. There was nothing to be concerned with on his form and he mentioned again on the form that he got regular massage treatments and was looking for an all over, relaxing massage. I cannot stress enough how normal all of this was! I did notice his address and the fact that he had travelled around 45 minutes to an hour to get to me. I suppose I should have asked about that, maybe, but what would he have said? It's not like he would have confessed that he doesn't have treatments with the same person because they probably never allowed him back after his first treatment or that no one in his area would see him any more. At the time, it just didn't strike me as odd. If he had given off a creepy vibe or made me feel uncomfortable, then maybe this amount of travel would have been more of a red flag to me, but he was perfectly nice and I didn't suspect a thing!

As always, I explained the treatment and how to get ready for the massage. Some practitioners insist that a Lomi Lomi massage requires the client to be completely naked due to the fact that the treatment is so focused on a relaxing flow over the whole body and is not carried out in sections. The therapist usually starts at the top of the head and chooses a side of the body to work down, keeping contact the whole time. The therapist will reach as far as he or she can without taking two steps and then flows back up the body. With this method, the therapist could be reaching from shoulder to toe in one motion and some would argue that any underwear just gets in the way. There is no set routine for a Lomi Lomi massage, and the treatment is carried out by instinct and what feels natural for that client, so you never know where you are going to next. The idea is that the client should feel like they are lying in the sea and the waves are flowing over them, the waves being the therapist's arms. However, especially with a male client, I do not agree with the client being completely naked, so I made sure to request that he kept his underwear on for the treatment. Again, he did not disagree with this or make any fuss so I did not think that there would be any funny business. Perhaps that was why I got so confused with what happened during the treatment!

I always start the treatment with the back of the body. He was lying face down with his arms down by his sides. He wasn't trying to move his arms or reach out to me or anything that would concern me or indicate that there was anything 'funny' going on, and the massage over the back of his body went by uneventfully. As this was a full body massage, I asked him to turn over so that I could work on the front of his body as well. As he was turning over, he mentioned that he had a lot of tension in his thighs, which I took to mean his quads, which were really tight. He asked if I could spend a bit more time in that area to ease the tension, and again, I never suspected a thing.

Lomi Lomi massage involves moving around the couch a lot and sometimes working both legs at the same time, so I was frequently flowing from one side to the other, continuing this wave-like flow. I had changed sides a few times and I was just working my way back around the couch again when he suddenly said, "Oh, I'm close to the edge."

I literally looked down at him and the couch and said, "But you're not going to fall off, you have space on both sides. You won't fall off."

He repeated, "No, no. I'm close to the edge."

I looked at him again and said, "But you're not going to fall off. There is space on the couch."

He kept repeating it, slightly more urgently and slowly, "No, I'm close to the edge."

But I just couldn't understand him. I kept trying to reason with him and reassure him that he was perfectly safe, but he kept insisting that he was close to the edge.

"I don't understand," I said, completely confused. "You're not going to fall. You have ample space each side of the couch, your head is not overhanging one end, your legs are not off the other end, you're not going to fall – you are perfectly fine!"

"Oh no, no, no. I'm close to the edge you know, like erm…"

"Like, erm, what? You won't fall!" I was getting a bit annoyed that he was interrupting the flow of the treatment and I kept thinking, what is wrong with you? You're not falling off a cliff. You're not going to die. What do you mean?

He continued, "No, no, no, like erm…"

Clarity started to strike me. Oh, here we go, I thought, starting to finally catch on.

"I'm going to come," he blurted out.

"Okay, your treatment is over," I said, backing off. "Get your stuff together. I'm out," and I started to leave the room. There had been absolutely no signs before that, I hadn't even noticed any bulges or raising of the towels that were covering his bits. I had absolutely no idea what he had been getting at! As I was leaving the room (I even had the door open), he shouted after me, "No, look at me!" and lifted up his towel to show me his penis and started to jerk himself off! At that, I couldn't leave the room fast enough!

I was working in a building with other businesses in and I ran upstairs, actually a few flights of stairs, and I was pretty out of breath when I got to my friend's floor. My friend was an IT guy and I knew he was working that day, thank God! I burst into his office and told him what was going on and asked if he could help me get this guy out of the building! I should mention here that my friend is over six foot and well built, and had told me before that if anything dodgy ever happened, he would be my bouncer!

I was a bit out of breath having run up the stairs, so I lingered at the top of the stairs to catch my breath and to this day I am not sure exactly how my 'bouncer' got the guy out of the building. When I came back down to my room there were used tissues everywhere, all over my massage couch and the floor where he had clearly finished himself off!

Obviously, I double gloved and grabbed a fresh tissue to pick everything up and throw it all out. My friend came back into the room after having got rid of the creepy client and told me that he wanted to book in again!

I was stunned! I shook my head violently and said, "Oh no, no, no…"

"That's what I thought," my friend said. "I've got rid of him for you and told him not to come back."

I am so thankful that he was in his office that day to help me out. I'm not sure what I would have done otherwise.

Unsurprisingly, I no longer offer Lomi Lomi massage to male clients!

Noisy Neighbours

I joined forces with a few therapist friends and for a short while, we offered treatments at a couple of big hotels in the village near where we lived. The two hotels did not have their own spa facilities but had a lot of clients who were looking to have treatments alongside their stay. We offered treatments in the hotel rooms. The hotel guest would ask the hotel for the treatments and the hotel would contact us, so until we arrived and got set up for our treatments, we wouldn't have a clue who our client was or exactly what their needs were. It was full on, exhausting, challenging at times and often quite fun. For the most part, clients were lovely, and the tips were always good!

We had been asked to do a couples' treatment but only I was available, so the clients were having to have a full body massage each, one after the other. They seemed to be happy with this, but the reception had told the guests that they could stay in the hotel room while the other was being treated. I always find this really uncomfortable and would prefer not to have an audience for my treatments! I arrived and started setting up in the client's room. As I was setting my bed up, I asked for them to each fill out a consultation form and decide who was going to have their treatment first. The guy asked if it was OK to stay in the room during each other's treatments and I agreed that it was alright but might be more relaxing if they waited at the bar or lounge. Without really conferring with his wife, he said, "Oh you can go first, and I'll stay here."

I couldn't tell if she minded or not. She specifically asked me for a relaxing full body massage and gently reminded her husband to stay quiet.

He lounged across the bed while I started his wife's full body massage. I focused in on her treatment and managed to block him out for the moment. Then he turned the TV on which was just by my head. His wife let out a long sigh but didn't say anything, so I shot him a look. "Oh sorry," he said and turned the volume down but left the TV on. I tried to zone out the TV and carry on with the treatment. I managed to get through the back massage and start on the backs of her legs when his phone rang, which he answered!

From his response, I got the impression that it was possibly a work-related call. He was very loud and had a demanding tone. Very calmly, his wife sighed again and said, "Darling, perhaps you should take that at the bar." He apologised to her, told whoever was on the other end that he needed to go and turned the TV volume back up.

I asked my client to turn over so I could continue her massage on the front of her body. As she turned over, she looked across at her husband. "Do you think you could turn the TV off, darling? I am trying to relax," she said, with very little of her original patience.

"Oh, yes dear," he said, leaning forward and flicking the TV off. He grabbed a book and started reading instead. My client let out a sigh and threw her head back down on the couch. There was only fifteen to twenty minutes left of her treatment time but I felt so bad for her that she hadn't been able to relax. I carried on the massage a little longer than I should have and included a bit of a scalp massage for her to try and help her to relax more, at which point her husband opened a packet of crisps and started crackling his way through those, very noisily. Her eyes snapped open, and she stared up at me. I tried an apologetic smile, and she forced a smile back at me. I brought the treatment to a very awkward end and she leapt off the couch, curtly thanked me, and stalked into the bathroom.

As I was swapping towels over, her husband snapped his book closed, jumped up off the bed and loudly proclaimed, "Right, my turn, then?"

I told him that it would take me a moment to swap the towels over and asked if he could get himself ready for his treatment in a robe, the same as his wife had done. I could hear the shower running in the bathroom, but seemingly oblivious to both the shower and his wife's displeasure at him, he barged into the bathroom to get changed. I did not hear exactly what was said but he was in there a while and she did most of the talking.

I stood next to my couch and awkwardly looked around for a distraction. After some time, he came out in his robe and asked if I needed a break or if I was ready for him. I said that I was fine and asked him to lie face down on the couch. I explained the treatment – full body massage, working both the back and front of the body…

He sank right into the couch and started breathing deeply before I had even started. Not long after I started working on his back, his wife came out of the bathroom and said, "I will be in the lounge so that you can enjoy your massage." She stalked out before she got an answer and her husband said, "Oops, I'm in trouble," and giggled boyishly.

I continued his massage, inwardly thinking he was a selfish dick and outwardly forcing calm and compassion.

I would say I was about fifteen minutes into an hour-and-fifteen-minute massage when the couple staying in the room above came back from wherever they had been and noisily slammed doors, threw shoes off and stomped across the floor. I tried turning the gentle music up a bit but there was not much more volume to give. Another door slammed and the bed loudly squeaked from someone throwing themselves on to it. Another loud squeak and a giggle, as clearly the other person flung themselves at the bed as well. My client seemed not to notice and was breathing very loudly. I wasn't sure if he was even awake.

I continued the back massage as the giggling continued. I tried to ignore it; these treatments were turning out a little more challenging than most. After a while the giggling stopped, and I breathed a sigh of relief. But then the bed started squeaking, rhythmically.

I realised my client was awake when he let out a barely concealed giggle. The couple upstairs were now really going at it, moaning, shouting, agreeing a lot. The bed sounded like it was being turned into kindling and the headboard had started smacking into the wall as well. Just in case there wasn't enough noise already! I didn't know what else to do, so I just kept massaging. I finished working on his back and then started massaging the back of his legs. He intermittently snored and giggled. It was all very confusing and uncomfortable. The couple upstairs just kept on going, getting louder and more vigorous as she agreed more readily with him. I wasn't sure if I should laugh or cry at this point.

It felt like the longest leg massage I had ever done. When I finally finished the back of his body, I gently said to him, "Are you ready to turn over?"

He took a deep breath then carefully and deliberately placed one hand at a time on the top corners of the couch, pushed himself into a plank position, looked deliberately down at his crotch, sighed and said, "No, I don't think that's a good idea." He let his knees drop but kept himself slightly pushed away from the couch, still staring down at himself. He sort of giggled again, looked up at the ceiling, looked at me, smiled and said, "I think we can leave it there."

I asked him if he would like me to leave the room so he could get off the couch and he slowly nodded and said, "I think that's best."

I left the room and when I heard the bathroom door shut, I let myself back in and called through, "I'll just tidy all my things and leave you in peace." The bathroom door opened a tiny crack, and a £20 note was poked through the gap. "I think you earned this today, thank you very much," he said. I took the money and he shut the bathroom door.

I put all my things away, turned off the music and headed out of the door. The couple upstairs were still going at it. I swear that bed must have been broken by the end.

As I was leaving the hotel, I passed through the lounge. My client's wife was sitting with a pot of tea. She started to look up as I was walking past. I felt my cheeks flushing red and I put my head down and hurried past. I was so embarrassed I couldn't bring myself to look her in the eye.

Acknowledgements

My dearest friend Susie Mackie, you are my inspiration. Without you, this book would still be a fanciful dream of mine. You are a truly unique and wonderful woman, and I am honoured to have you as a friend. Your guidance and stunning example with your book *Women of Spirit* has given me the push that I needed to write my own collection. I will forever be grateful.

Karen Poyzer, Laura Tinney, Vicky James, Zoe Hinkley, Laura Scott and every therapist who has chosen to remain anonymous, a thousand thank yous for taking the time to share your stories with me and giving me your blessings to write and publish your crazy memories! It has been an absolute pleasure and of course, this book couldn't exist without your input.

Finally, a truly heartfelt thanks to my amazing partner Silviu, without whom I would not have the courage to be my authentic self, or the self-belief to even attempt to publish a book. All my love.

Kayleigh

Lightning Source UK Ltd.
Milton Keynes UK
UKHW010623291021
393035UK00001B/178